T0259194

Update on Ankle Arthritis

Guest Editors

ALAN R. CATANZARITI, DPM, FACFAS
ROBERT W. MENDICINO, DPM, FACFAS

CLINICS IN PODIATRIC MEDICINE AND SURGERY

www.podiatric.theclinics.com

Consulting Editor

THOMAS ZGONIS, DPM, FACFAS

April 2009 • Volume 26 • Number 2

SAUNDERS an imprint of ELSEVIER, Inc.

W.B. SAUNDERS COMPANY
A Division of Elsevier Inc.

1600 John F. Kennedy Boulevard ● Suite 1800 ● Philadelphia, Pennsylvania 19103-2899

http://www.theclinics.com

CLINICS IN PODIATRIC MEDICINE AND SURGERY Volume 26, Number 2
April 2009 ISSN 0891-8422, ISBN-13: 978-1-4377-0531-7, ISBN-10: 1-4377-0531-6

Editor: Patrick Manley
Developmental Editor: Donald Mumford

© 2009 Elsevier ■ All rights reserved.

This journal and the individual contributions contained in it are protected under copyright by Elsevier, and the following terms and conditions apply to their use:

Photocopying
Single photocopies of single articles may be made for personal use as allowed by national copyright laws. Permission of the Publisher and payment of a fee is required for all other photocopying, including multiple or systematic copying, copying for advertising or promotional purposes, resale, and all forms of document delivery. Special rates are available for educational institutions that wish to make photocopies for non-profit educational classroom use. For information on how to seek permission visit www.elsevier.com/permissions or call: (+44) 1865 843830 (UK)/(+1) 215 239 3804 (USA).

Derivative Works
Subscribers may reproduce tables of contents or prepare lists of articles including abstracts for internal circulation within their institutions. Permission of the Publisher is required for resale or distribution outside the institution. Permission of the Publisher is required for all other derivative works, including compilations and translations (please consult www.elsevier.com/permissions).

Electronic Storage or Usage
Permission of the Publisher is required to store or use electronically any material contained in this journal, including any article or part of an article (please consult www.elsevier.com/permissions). Except as outlined above, no part of this publication may be reproduced, stored in a retrieval system or transmitted in any form or by any means, electronic, mechanical, photocopying, recording or otherwise, without prior written permission of the Publisher.

Notice
No responsibility is assumed by the Publisher for any injury and/or damage to persons or property as a matter of products liability, negligence or otherwise, or from any use or operation of any methods, products, instructions or ideas contained in the material herein. Because of rapid advances in the medical sciences, in particular, independent verification of diagnoses and drug dosages should be made.

Although all advertising material is expected to conform to ethical (medical) standards, inclusion in this publication does not constitute a guarantee or endorsement of the quality or value of such product or of the claims made of it by its manufacturer.

Clinics in Podiatric Medicine and Surgery (ISSN 0891-8422) is published quarterly by Elsevier Inc., 360 Park Avenue South, New York, NY 10010-1710. Months of publication are January, April, July, and October. Business and Editorial Offices: 1600 John F. Kennedy Blvd., Suite 1800, Philadelphia, PA 191023-2899. Customer Service Office: 6277 Sea Harbor Drive, Orlando, FL 32887-4800. Periodicals postage paid at New York, NY, and additional mailing offices. Subscription prices are $229.00 per year for US individuals, $360.00 per year for US institutions, $118.00 per year for US students and residents, $275.00 per year for Canadian individuals, $445.00 for Canadian institutions, $326.00 for international individuals, $445.00 per year for international institutions and $167.00 per year for Canadian and foreign students/residents. To receive student/resident rate, orders must be accompanied by name of affiliated institution, date of term, and the *signature* of program/residency coordinator on institution letterhead. Orders will be billed at individual rate until proof of status is received. Foreign air speed delivery is included in all *Clinics* subscription prices. All prices are subject to change without notice. POSTMASTER: Send address changes to *Clinics in Podiatric Medicine and Surgery*, Elsevier Periodicals Customer Service, 6277 Sea Harbor Drive, Orlando, FL 32887-4800. **Customer Service: 1-800-654-2452 (US). From outside of the US, call 314-453-7041. Fax: 314-453-5170. E-mail: JournalsCustomerService-usa@ elsevier.com (for print support); JournalsOnlineSupport-usa@elsevier.com (for online support).**

Reprints. For copies of 100 or more of articles in this publication, please contact the Commercial Reprints Department, Elsevier Inc., 360 Park Avenue South, New York, NY 10010-1710. Tel.: 212-633-3812; Fax: 212-462-1935; E-mail: reprints@elsevier.com.

Clinics in Podiatric Medicine and Surgery is covered in *MEDLINE/PubMed (Index Medicus)* and *EMBASE/Excerpta Medica.*

Printed and bound by CPI Group (UK) Ltd, Croydon, CR0 4YY

Transferred to Digital Print 2011

CLINICS IN PODIATRIC MEDICINE AND SURGERY

CONSULTING EDITOR
THOMAS ZGONIS, DPM, FACFAS

EDITORIAL BOARD MEMBERS – USA

Babak Baravarian, DPM, FACFAS
Neal M Blitz, DPM, FACFAS
Peter A Blume, DPM, FACFAS
Patrick R Burns, DPM, FACFAS
Alan R Catanzariti, DPM, FACFAS
Luke D Cicchinelli, DPM, FACFAS
Lawrence A DiDomenico, DPM, FACFAS
Lawrence Ford, DPM, FACFAS
Robert G Frykberg, DPM
Jordan P Grossman, DPM, FACFAS
Graham A Hamilton, DPM, FACFAS
Allen M Jacobs, DPM, FACFAS
Gary Peter Jolly, DPM, FACFAS
Molly S Judge, DPM, FACFAS
Adam S Landsman, DPM, PhD, FACFAS
Vincent J Mandracchia, DPM, MHA, FACFAS
Luis E Marin, DPM, FACFAS
Robert W Mendicino, DPM, FACFAS
Samuel S Mendicino, DPM, FACFAS
Thomas S Roukis, DPM, PhD, FACFAS
Laurence G Rubin, DPM, FACFAS
John M Schuberth, DPM
John J Stapleton, DPM, AACFAS
Trent K Statler, DPM, FACFAS
Jerome K Steck, DPM, FACFAS
John S Steinberg, DPM, FACFAS
George F Wallace, DPM, FACFAS
Bruce Werber, DPM, FACFAS
Glenn M Weinraub, DPM, FACFAS
Charles M Zelen, DPM, FACFAS

EDITORIAL BOARD MEMBERS – INTERNATIONAL

Thanos Badekas, MD (Athens, Greece)
Tanil Esemenli, MD (Istanbul, Turkey)
Armin Koller, MD (Muenster, Germany)
Ali Oznur, MD (Ankara, Turkey)
Enrico Parino, MD (Torino, Italy)
Pier Carlo Pisani, MD (Torino, Italy)
Vasilios D Polyzois, MD, PhD, FHCOS (Athens, Greece)
Emmanouil D Stamatis, MD, FHCOS, FACS (Athens, Greece)
Victor Valderrabano, MD, PhD (Basel, Switzerland)

Contributors

CONSULTING EDITOR

THOMAS ZGONIS, DPM, FACFAS
Associate Professor, Department of Orthopaedics; Chief, Division of Podiatric Medicine
and Surgery; Director, Podiatric Surgical Residency and Fellowship Programs, The
University of Texas Health Science Center at San Antonio, San Antonio, Texas

GUEST EDITORS

ALAN R. CATANZARITI, DPM, FACFAS
Director of Residency Training, Department of Foot and Ankle Surgery, The Western
Pennsylvania Hospital, Pittsburgh, Pennsylvania

ROBERT W. MENDICINO, DPM, FACFAS
Chairman, Department of Foot and Ankle Surgery, The Western Pennsylvania Hospital,
Pittsburgh, Pennsylvania

AUTHORS

JASON B. ANDERSON, DPM
Foot & Ankle Fellow, Jewish Hospital, University of Louisville, Louisville, Kentucky

RONALD BELCZYK, DPM
Clinical Instructor, Department of Orthopaedics; Fellow, Reconstructive Foot and Ankle
Surgery, Division of Podiatric Medicine and Surgery, The University of Texas Health
Science Center at San Antonio, San Antonio, Texas

FRANK BONGIOVANNI, DPM, C. Ped
Attending Physician, Weil Foot and Ankle Institute, Des Plaines, Illinois

CODY A. BOWERS, DPM
Resident, Department of Foot and Ankle Surgery, The Western Pennsylvania Hospital,
Pittsburgh, Pennsylvania

ALAN R. CATANZARITI, DPM, FACFAS
Director of Residency Training, Department of Foot and Ankle Surgery, The Western
Pennsylvania Hospital, Pittsburgh, Pennsylvania

THOMAS J. CHANG, DPM
Northern California Foot and Ankle Center

MONIQUE GOURDINE-SHAW, DPM
Lieutenant Commander, Medical Service Corps., United States Navy, United States Naval
Academy, Annapolis; Veterans Affairs Maryland Healthcare Center, Baltimore, Maryland

KIRK A. GROGAN, DPM
Northern California Foot and Ankle Center

JORDAN P. GROSSMAN, DPM, FACFAS
Director of Podiatric Medicine Training, St. Vincent Charity Hospital, Cleveland, Ohio

SHINE JOHN, DPM
Surgical Fellow, Weil Foot and Ankle Institute, Des Plaines, Illinois

ROBERT MICHAEL JOSEPH, DPM, PhD
Clinical Research Associate, Center for Tissue Regeneration and Engineering at Dayton, University of Dayton, Dayton, Ohio

CHUL KIM, DPM
Chief Resident, Department of Foot and Ankle Surgery, The Western Pennsylvania Hospital, Pittsburgh, Pennsylvania

ANDREW J. KLUESNER, DPM
Third-Year Foot and Ankle Surgery Resident, Department of Podiatric Surgery, University of Pittsburgh Medical Center, South Side Hospital, Pittsburgh, Pennsylvania

BRADLEY M. LAMM, DPM
Head of the Podiatry Section, International Center for Limb Lengthening, Rubin Institute for Advanced Orthopedics, Sinai Hospital of Baltimore, Baltimore, Maryland

MICHAEL S. LEE, DPM, FACFAS
Associate Clinical Professor, College of Podiatric Medicine and Surgery, Des Moines University, Des Moines; Foot and Ankle Surgery, Capital Orthopaedics and Sports Medicine, Des Moines, Iowa

MICHAEL C. LYONS II, DPM
Third Year Resident, St. Vincent Charity Hospital, Cleveland, Ohio

ROBERT W. MENDICINO, DPM, FACFAS
Chairman, Department of Foot and Ankle Surgery, The Western Pennsylvania Hospital, Pittsburgh, Pennsylvania

DAVID M. MILLWARD, BS
Student, College of Podiatric Medicine and Surgery, Des Moines University, Des Moines, Iowa

VASILIOS D. POLYZOIS, MD, PhD
Chief of Orthopaedic Traumatology, KAT General Hospital, Athens, Greece

SHANNON M. RUSH, DPM, FACFAS
Camino Division, Department of Orthopedics, Palo Alto Medical Foundation, Mountain View, California

ROBERT S. SALK, DPM
Northern California Foot and Ankle Center

JOHN J. STAPLETON, DPM
Associate, VSAS Orthopaedics, Allentown; Clinical Assistant Professor, Department of Surgery, Penn State College of Medicine, Hershey, Pennsylvania

JEROME K. STECK, DPM, FACFAS
Southern Arizona Orthopedics; Assistant Clinical Professor of Surgery, University of Arizona, Tucson, Arizona; Attending Faculty, Jewish Hospital, University of Louisville, Louisville, Kentucky

DANE K. WUKICH, MD
Assistant Professor, Department of Orthopedic Surgery, University of Pittsburgh, Pittsburgh; Chief, Division of Foot and Ankle Surgery, Department of Orthopedic Surgery, University of Pittsburgh, Pittsburgh; Director, Comprehensive Foot and Ankle Center, University of Pittsburgh Medical Center, Pittsburgh, Pennsylvania

THOMAS ZGONIS, DPM, FACFAS
Associate Professor, Department of Orthopaedics; Chief, Division of Podiatric Medicine and Surgery; Director, Podiatric Surgical Residency and Fellowship Programs, The University of Texas Health Science Center at San Antonio, San Antonio, Texas

Contents

> Trends in science are beginning to suggest that cartilage degeneration may be related to a chronic imbalance in extracellular matrix metabolism. In cartilage, a combination of biomechanical, biochemical, and matrix-related signaling pathways regulates the equilibrium between cartilage anabolism and catabolism. A potential limitation of many current treatments of osteoarthritis is that they may not comprehensively restore regulation of a balance between cartilage anabolism and catabolism.

> Ankle joint distraction has been shown to be a viable alternative to ankle arthrodesis or ankle replacement. The authors' approach to ankle joint preservation includes articulated ankle joint distraction, resection of blocking osteophytes, release of muscle and joint contractures, and realignment osseous ankle procedures. In a previous study that used this technique, 78% of patients maintained their ankle range of motion and had none to occasional moderate pain that could be managed generally with nonsteroid anti-inflammatory drugs alone. The rationale as to why joint distraction is successful is largely unknown. Therefore, the purpose of this study was to evaluate pre- and postoperative ankle MRI scans of patients who underwent hinged ankle joint distraction with external fixation.

> Management of ankle arthritis can be difficult for the physician and patient. Conservative options are limited but should be exhausted in an effort to prolong ankle arthrodesis. Custom braces can provide an effective means

its ideal indication. Current literature does support its use in the treatment of ankle arthritis, however.

THE CLINICS ARE NOW AVAILABLE ONLINE!

Access your subscription at:
www.theclinics.com

Foreword

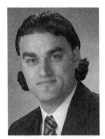

Thomas Zgonis, DPM, FACFAS
Consulting Editor

Ankle arthritis is a frequent debilitating condition and most commonly affects the younger patient as a result of trauma. Traumatic injuries may be the leading cause of degenerative changes within the ankle joint but other contributing factors such as an inflammatory, infectious, or neuropathic arthropathy can also lead to persistent pain and deterioration of the ankle joint. Primary "idiopathic" osteoarthritis is less commonly encountered as compared to the hip or knee but is becoming more prevalent among our growing elderly population.

This issue is dedicated to the advancement of conservative and surgical treatments of ankle arthritis. Current surgical treatment options for the end stage ankle arthritis remain between an ankle arthrodesis and an endoprosthesis procedure. This issue elaborates on some of the technical considerations in performing an ankle arthrodesis or total ankle joint replacement, along with appropriate patient selection for each procedure. During the last decade, it has been very exciting to witness the major advances in total ankle arthroplasty along with the various implant designs that have become available in the United States. In addition, this issue will also cover some of the current concepts and techniques that are offering some promising results in delaying the need for a joint arthrodesis and/or replacement.

These novel techniques are described as an alternative to a joint destructive procedure and have been paramount to the treating surgeon's armamentarium. Examples of these procedures which have been reported in the recent literature include but are not limited to the ankle distraction arthroplasty, lower extremity osteotomies to address the ankle pathomechanics and talar resurfacing with new advances in cartilage repair. Attention is given not only to the advantages but also to some of the pitfalls of these newer procedures.

The constant advancement in technology, research and surgeon training has provided us with many different options to address the painful and debilitating symptoms associated with the end stage ankle arthritis. The Guest Editors in this issue, Dr. Catanzariti and Dr. Mendicino, have done an outstanding job in addressing some of the most common etiologies and pathomechanics that lead to an ankle arthritis, along with the various treatment options and successful outcomes. Their knowledge

Clin Podiatr Med Surg 26 (2009) xv–xvi
doi:10.1016/j.cpm.2009.02.002
0891-8422/09/$ – see front matter © 2009 Elsevier Inc. All rights reserved.

podiatric.theclinics.com

and expertise on this subject is well known through their numerous publications and contributions to our profession. Lastly, a great thank you to all of the contributors and editorial board members for their continuous efforts and commitment to the *Clinics in Podiatric Medicine and Surgery*.

Thomas Zgonis, DPM, FACFAS
The University of Texas Health Science Center at San Antonio
7703 Floyd Curl Drive, MSC 7776
San Antonio, TX 78229, USA

E-mail address:
zgonis@uthscsa.edu (T. Zgonis)

Preface

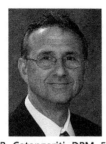 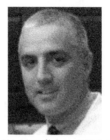

Alan R. Catanzariti, DPM, FACFAS   Robert W. Mendicino, DPM, FACFAS
Guest Editors

Arthritis is the leading cause of disability in the United States. People diagnosed with degenerative joint disease of the ankle constitute a large number of patients who experience pain and disability. This issue of *Clinics in Podiatric Medicine and Surgery* is dedicated to management of ankle arthritis. It is our pleasure to serve as Guest Editors.

The articles published in this issue have been authored by a diverse group of foot and ankle surgeons from various geographic areas. The first article by Robert Joseph, DPM provides an overview of basic science as it applies to osteoarthritis and provides insight into future technologies that might be available for cartilage replacement. The next article by Drs. John and Bongiovanni discuss the use of lower extremity braces to manage ankle deformity and instability. Dr. Chang's article describes the use of viscosupplementation to manage ankle arthritis. The following article by Drs. Grossman and Lyons provides a comprehensive review of osteochondral lesions of the talus. Drs. Kluesner and Wukich introduce arthrodiastasis as a joint sparing procedure for degenerative joint disease of the ankle. This is followed by an article authored by Drs. Lamm and Gourdin-Shaw describing the use of magnetic resonance imaging to evaluate ankle distraction. The article by Dr. Rush reviews the implications of malalignment on ankle arthritis and the role of supramalleolar osteotomies to address underlying deformity. The next three articles focus on fusion procedures including traditional ankle arthrodesis (Drs. Bowers, Mendicino, and Catanzariti), arthroscopic ankle arthrodesis (Dr. Lee), and tibiotalocalcaneal arthrodesis (Drs. Kim, Mendicino, and Catanzariti). The final article, authored by Dr. Steck, on total ankle replacement focuses on potential complications.

There are many people who deserve thanks for the preparation of this issue, most importantly, our families. A special thanks to our contributing editors for their hard work and dedication that made this issue possible. Lastly, we would like to thank the West

Clin Podiatr Med Surg 26 (2009) xvii–xviii
doi:10.1016/j.cpm.2009.03.003
0891-8422/09/$ – see front matter © 2009 Elsevier Inc. All rights reserved.

Penn Allegheny Health System for their support of graduate medical education and academics.

We hope you enjoy reading this issue of Clinics.

Alan R. Catanzariti, DPM, FACFAS
Director of Residency Training
Department of Foot and Ankle Surgery
The Western Pennsylvania Hospital

Robert W. Mendicino, DPM, FACFAS
Chair, Department of Foot and Ankle Surgery
The Western Pennsylvania Hospital

E-mail addresses:
acatanzariti@faiwp.com (A.R. Catanzariti)
rmendicino@faiwp.com (R.W. Mendicino)

Osteoarthritis of the Ankle: Bridging Concepts in Basic Science with Clinical Care

Robert Michael Joseph, DPM, PhD

KEYWORDS

- Cartilage • Metabolism • Homeostasis
- Metabolic stress raiser • Osteoarthritis • Cartilage degeneration

Osteoarthritis (OA) is a condition affecting more than 20 million Americans that results in joint pain, dysfunction, and disability.[1] The prevalence of OA is estimated at 125 per 1000 persons.[2] OA is a leading cause of lost wages in the United States, and more than 80% of the population older than 75 years present with symptoms of OA.[3] Domestic estimated costs of OA exceed $60 billion annually, and cumulative social, economic, and medical costs were estimated to be 1.1% of the gross national product in 1999.[1,3,4] Although ankle OA only represents 1% of arthritic joints, studies suggest that the physical, emotional, and functional pain and limitation of end-stage ankle arthritis equal or exceed those of OA of the hip and that ankle OA can be as incapacitating as end-stage kidney disease and congestive heart failure.[1,4,5]

Regardless of which joint(s) are affected by OA, the preeminent clinical challenges to OA remain reduction of pain and restoration of joint function. Clinical treatment of OA is hampered by medical science's current inability to reverse or prevent hyaline cartilage degeneration from joint surfaces despite pharmacologic, viscosupplementing, arthroscopic, and cell transplantation therapies. As we enter an era of regenerative medicine, our growing capacity to understand and manipulate the physiologic, developmental, and biomechanical properties of tissues further brings us closer to tissue regeneration.

Trends in science are beginning to suggest that some chronic progressive degenerative conditions are related to a chronic metabolic imbalance of the tissues, and cartilage is no exception.[6–10] A growing number of studies suggest that pathways of chronic cartilage degeneration might best be understood as an imbalance in cartilage metabolism, whereby cartilage catabolism (degradation) exceeds cartilage anabolism (growth

Center for Tissue Regeneration and Engineering at Dayton, University of Dayton, 305 Oakwood Avenue, Dayton, OH 45409, USA
E-mail address: footbiochemistry@hotmail.com

Clin Podiatr Med Surg 26 (2009) 169–184
doi:10.1016/j.cpm.2008.12.005
0891-8422/08/$ – see front matter © 2009 Elsevier Inc. All rights reserved.

and repair) in a manner consistent with OA.[11] Hence, the scientific and medical challenge for successful long-term treatment of OA may be restoration of the metabolic equilibrium between anabolism and catabolism.[11] The temporizing nature of current treatments of OA may be a consequence of incomplete restoration of a metabolic equilibrium between states of cartilage degeneration and repair. As our knowledge of cartilage biology expands, so does an appreciation that there are unique physiologic and biomechanical properties of ankle cartilage that influence function, form, metabolism, and the subsequent capacity to treat ankle arthritis, with an ultimate goal of cartilage repair, regeneration, and engineering. Science has come to appreciate that cartilage is a dynamic tissue whose mechanical properties and biologic activity are intimately regulated through biochemical signaling and biophysical forces of compression, shear, and fluid flow. This review attempts to relate scientific advancements in our understanding of ankle cartilage's unique properties with the potential challenges of current treatments and the direction of future treatment.

GENERAL COMPOSITION AND FUNCTION OF CARTILAGE

Weight-bearing activities can transmit forces up to 10 times a person's body weight through the joints of the lower extremity.[12] Cartilage's shock-absorbing properties are responsible for dissipating many of these forces.[12] Cartilage uses synovial fluid, an ultrafiltrate of blood, for transport of nutrients and elimination of metabolic wastes rather than an organized vascular system of arterioles and capillaries. Processes of diffusion and fluid flow dynamics from weight-bearing activity regulate metabolite transport to and from cartilage through synovial fluid.[13] Water comprises 65% to 80% of cartilage weight, with the remaining 20% principally consisting of extracellular matrix (ECM) composed of various collagens, proteoglycan (PG), and glycosaminoglycan.[12] The ECM is grossly organized as a scaffold of collagens that provide an infrastructure for PG organization and retention of water. Collagen retains PG within cartilage through frictional and electrostatic interactions.[12] Negatively charged PGs retain water within the cartilage matrix through electrostatic interactions.[12] PG helps to dissipate joint forces by electrostatic resistance to biomechanical displacement of water from the cartilage matrix when weight-bearing forces of compression, ploughing, and sheer are applied to joints.[12] As cartilage experiences biomechanical loads, water is expressed from cartilage matrix much like water is expressed from a sponge under pressure. Degradation and loss of PG from cartilage are related to cartilage softening and loss of the shock-absorbing properties of cartilage. PG loss from cartilage is preceded by collagen fiber degradation in the early stages of OA. Collagen degradation exposes PG to degradative enzymes that further promote cartilage degeneration.

Extracellular Matrix in General

Cartilage histology can be grossly characterized in layers by superficial, middle, and deep zones, with the superficial zone being closest to the joint space and comprising 10% to 20% of cartilage thickness and the deep zone abutting subchondral bone and comprising 30% to 40% of cartilage thickness (**Fig. 1**).[12,14] The middle zone is between the superficial and deep zones. Matrix surrounding chondrocytes is circumferentially characterized as pericellular, territorial, and interterritorial regions (see **Fig. 1**).[14] These zones and regions have unique cellular, compositional, and biomechanical properties. The heterogeneous nature and complexity of cellular and matrix organization throughout cartilage make cartilage a difficult tissue to regenerate in vivo and to engineer ex vivo.

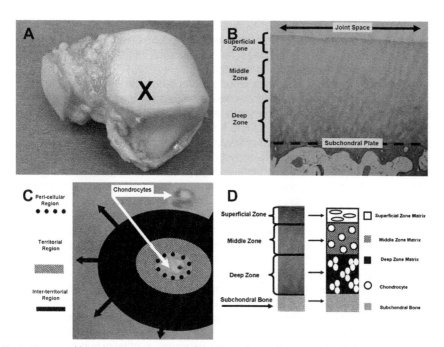

Fig. 1. Gross and histologic appearance of cartilage from a human talus. (*A*) Nondegenerated articular cartilage of the talus. "X" marks the region of the talar dome, from which an osteochondral sample was harvested for histologic examination, as demonstrated in *B*, *D*. (*B*) Hematoxylin and eosin staining of cartilage demonstrates organization of cartilage into superficial, middle, and deep zones. The superficial zone is closest to the joint space. The deep zone is closest to subchondral bone. (*C*) General illustration demonstrates circumferential classification of regions of matrix surrounding a chondrocyte. (*D*) General illustration relates talus histology to diagrams of cartilage. Note a distinction in matrix composition among cartilage zones. Note a distinction in the shape (morphology) of chondrocytes represented in each zone.

One compositional difference among zones and regions of cartilage is the distribution of PG.[15] There are multiple PGs in cartilage, with aggrecan being the largest and most significant shock-absorbing PG.[12] Aggrecan content is greatest in the middle zone and lowest in the superficial zone of cartilage.[16,17] The superficial zone of cartilage tends to have smaller aggregates of PG than the deeper zones.[12,16,18] The superficial zone has the greatest tensile properties of all three zones; high-tensile properties are attributed to the parallel orientation of collagen fibers with the joint surface.[19,20] Collagen fibers of the superficial zone are of smaller diameter than those of deeper zones.[14] Levels of aggrecan double in the pericellular regions in comparison to the interterritorial regions.[12,16,18] Gradients of PG content throughout zones have profound affects on the shock-absorbing properties of cartilage, because PG content in cartilage directly influences cartilage stiffness and shock-absorbing properties. Higher PG content is directly related to greater modulus and stiffness and lower hydraulic permeability, whereas lower PG content is associated with softening of cartilage and reduced shock absorption.[21] PG gradients potentially cause nonuniform deformation properties throughout cartilage and contribute to the complexity of modeling cartilage deformation under joint-loading conditions.

Clinically resurfacing or filling cartilage voids with biologic or synthetic implants that do not replicate the complex deformation properties of native cartilage is disadvantaged in stimulating durable cartilage repair, because mechanical forces directly influence cartilage homeostasis and function.[22,23]

A second compositional difference among zones is that some matrix molecules are not found in all zones. Superficial zone protein is an example of a small glycoprotein isolated to the superficial zone and only synthesized by chondrocytes from the superficial zone and synovial cells.[24,25] Its exact role in matrix organization and cartilage homeostasis is unknown, but sequence homology with megakaryocyte-stimulating factor precursor suggests a cytoprotective and lubricating role in cartilage that limits invasive cell adhesion to cartilage surfaces.[26] Interestingly, a defect in the gene encoding superficial zone protein is found in individuals with camptodactyly-arthropathy-coxa varapericarditis syndrome, a condition that causes early degeneration of large joints.[27]

Despite the limited content and isolation of some matrix molecules within specific cartilage zones, the physiologic significance of these molecules should not necessarily be relegated and unaccounted for in the development of matrix scaffold technology. A molecule's limited distribution within cartilage does not necessarily relate a limited role in cartilage repair or regeneration, as suggested in camptodactyly-arthropathy-coxa varapericarditis syndrome. The complicated nature of feedback, inhibitory, and amplifying signal transduction cascades potentially propagates focal biochemical events initiated by minor matrix components into systemic tissue responses.

Early selection of scaffold composites may have been just as related to practicality in choosing well-characterized and clinically approved synthetic materials, such as polyglycolic acid, rather than optimal biologic properties. Current scaffold designs do not incorporate smaller matrix constituents. Newer scaffold strategies are being developed, however, that use a layered scaffold approach incorporating greater matrix heterogeneity that is more similar to native cartilage.

Chondrocytes in General

Chondrocytes, the resident cells of cartilage, only make up 2% of the tissue volume.[14] There are fewer chondrocytes located in the deeper zones of cartilage than in the superficial zone.[12] Chondrocytes are principally responsible for maintaining the ECM through a delicate balance of anabolic and catabolic activities.[12] Sparse cellularity of cartilage makes chondrocytes responsible for a disproportionately large region of ECM in comparison to many tissues, a consequence that likely limits cartilage's ability for self-repair. The disproportionate ratio of matrix to cellularity also makes cartilage a tissue of relatively low metabolic activity. Hence, subtle changes in chondrocyte metabolism likely have a profound impact on matrix cartilage homeostasis and health. These conditions pose interesting challenges in the development of tissue regeneration constructs with regard to optimal parameters of construct cellularity and density. Because fetal cartilage has a greater cellular content than adult cartilage, it is unclear what the optimum numbers of cells are to meet the time-dependent requirements of regeneration, repair, and maintenance of new cartilage in an adult. Optimal cellular content and seeding density for cartilage regeneration constructs are currently unknown and likely depend on several construct factors, including cell type, matrix conditions, growth factor availability, and biomechanical loading conditions.

Cell Morphology in General

Difference in chondrocyte morphology is a distinguishing feature among cartilage zones. Cells residing in the superficial layers of cartilage are morphologically flatter than chondrocytes in deeper zones.[14] This has significant physiologic implications, because studies suggest that chondrocyte shape plays a regulatory role in cartilage metabolism.

Studies demonstrate that chondrocytes with flat morphology have a greater capacity for producing type I collagen than round chondrocytes.[28] When chondrocytes spread like fibroblasts in monolayer culture, they begin to synthesize type I collagen predominantly rather than the native type II collagen found in cartilage. They become more "fibroblast-like."[28] The same chondrocytes down-regulate type I collagen synthesis and up-regulate type II collagen synthesis after regaining a round morphology with enzymatic release of the cells from culture, hence returning to a more "chondrocyte-like" phenotype.[28] This phenomenon does not seem to be sensitive to cell interaction with several cartilage matrix components in vitro, thereby suggesting limited capacity of cartilage matrix molecules to stabilize chondrocyte shape and phenotype categorically. Isolated synthesis of superficial zone protein from flat chondrocytes also suggests that cell morphology may play a role in regulating matrix metabolism.[25]

Histologic studies of cartilage explants relate patterns of pericellular collagen organization that correlate with cell shape.[29] It is not clear whether matrix composition and organization act to stabilize or determine cell morphology. In any case, morphology is not the sole regulator of matrix metabolism, because the normal flat chondrocytes of the superficial zone continue to synthesize superficial zone protein when cultured in media that maintain a round chondrocyte morphology.[30]

Further research is needed to clarify how chondrocyte morphology and matrix metabolism influence each other. The regulatory relation between cell morphology and cell metabolism may potentially be manipulated in the future to improve the way in which chondrocytes are seeded and maintained in scaffolds.

REGULATORS OF CARTILAGE METABOLISM
Overview of Cytokine Regulation of Metabolism

Cytokines are bioactive molecules that affect cartilage metabolism through a combination of stimulatory and inhibitory pathways.[31] Some cytokines promote catabolic process in cartilage, whereas others promote anabolic pathways.[32] Cytokines mediate chondrocyte metabolism through autocrine, paracrine, and intracrine responses.[33] Cytokines have been shown to elicit metabolic responses directly through interaction with chondrocyte receptors and coordinately with ECM interactions with chondrocytes.[34,35] Chondrocyte response to cytokine stimulation has been shown to vary among chondrocyte populations from different zones.[30] Superficial zone chondrocytes are more sensitive to interleukin (IL)-1–stimulated catabolism and less affected by interleukin-1 receptor antagonist protein inhibition of IL-1 activities than chondrocytes from deeper zones.[30] Inflammatory cytokines, such as IL-1 and tumor necrosis factor (TNF), have been shown to promote cartilage degeneration by stimulating catabolic activities, such as increased metalloproteinase activity, and suppression of anabolic activities, such as PG synthesis.[36,37] Other cytokines, such as tissue growth factor (TGF) and insulin-like growth factor (IGF), stimulate anabolic processes that promote cartilage anabolism and repair, such as PG synthesis.[31]

Although IL-1–, TNF-, TGF-, and IGF-mediated activities have been extensively studied in cartilage, these are but a few of the many cytokines that act on cartilage through dependent and independent signal transduction pathways that are coordinately controlled by other cytokines, tissue biomechanics, and matrix interactions.[37] An example of coordinated signaling through cytokine and matrix molecule interaction with chondrocytes is TGFβ–mediated increase in PG synthesis when chondrocytes interact with type II collagen in vitro.[34] In vitro mechanical loading of cartilage explants has also been shown to modulate tissue response to cytokine stimulation.[33,34,38,39] Cross-regulatory pathways may potentially act to inhibit cartilage repair or synergistically promote cartilage anabolism and repair, such as the synergistic effects of IGF and osteogenic protein-1 on ECM synthesis in vitro.[40] Further understanding of the interrelations of coregulatory pathways of cytokine signaling is an integral part of developing strategies for cytokine-based treatments of OA.

Overview of Matrix Molecule Regulation of Metabolism

The ECM plays a vital role in cartilage homeostasis. The composition, organization, and structure of the ECM provide chondrocytes with cues regarding the general health of cartilage tissue. In healthy ankle cartilage, interactions between the ECM and chondrocytes likely promote a metabolic balance between cartilage anabolism and catabolism. Cadaver studies are consistent with steady-state balance of collagen synthesis with cartilage ageing.[41] Comparative studies between cadaver knee and ankle cartilage suggest that knee cartilage does not maintain the general state of metabolic equilibrium observed in ankle cartilage during aging.[41–44] It is unconfirmed albeit speculated that this metabolic difference between ankles and knees may contribute to a higher incidence of OA in knees than in ankles.[9,45]

In in vitro and in vivo studies, the metabolic equilibrium between cartilage anabolism and catabolism can be disrupted by matrix degradation products within joint synovial fluid and the cartilage matrix.[46] This disruption promotes cartilage degeneration resembling degeneration observed in OA.[46] Collagen, hyaluronan, and fibronectin are all cartilage matrix molecules whose degradation products promote cartilage degeneration.[9,46–48] Fibronectin fragments (Fnfs) have been most extensively studied in cartilage and promote cartilage degeneration by enhancing cartilage catabolism through up-regulation of metalloproteinase activities and suppressing cartilage anabolism through the suppression of PG synthesis.[9] It is suggested that accumulations of matrix degradation products in cartilage might promote cartilage degeneration by altering normal signaling of native matrix molecules.[46] Another possibility is that degradation products act through unique independent interactions with chondrocytes to promote cartilage degeneration.[46]

Overview of Biomechanical Force Regulation of Metabolism

Physiologic loading of joints is known to be vital in preserving joint health.[49–51] Disruption of normal joint-loading mechanics has been shown to predispose cartilage to degenerative process. This is clinically evident in posttraumatic and congenital deformity of the ankle, including ankle instability and procurvatum and recurvatum deformity.[50,52,53]

The mechanical properties of cartilage are complex and intimately related to cartilage matrix composition, which varies throughout zones of cartilage tissue.[54] This results in unique deformation properties of cartilage in each zone of cartilage, in addition to cartilage as a whole.[55]

Joint cartilage undergoes a combination of biomechanical forces that include compression, sheer, and ploughing. These forces have been shown to influence various elements of tissue homeostasis, including tissue differentiation, morphogenesis of cartilage layers, matrix homeostasis, and cell proliferation.[22,23,49,56–58] The exact mechanisms by which biomechanical forces regulate cartilage homeostasis are still unknown and complicated by experimental variations in tested tissues; culture conditions; and the loading parameters of load frequency, duration, and magnitude. A growing body of research suggests that dynamic compression stimulates more anabolic than catabolic activities, such as increased PG synthesis and reduced cell proliferation, compared with static compression, although there are reports that dynamic compression can promote physical weakening and breakdown of collagen.[59–61] Limited studies suggest that sheer forces may have a chondroprotective effect on cartilage in some circumstances.[23,62,63] These studies report sheer-related increase in collagen synthesis and synthesis of a chondroprotection molecule, PG-4.[23,62,63] Sheer forces have also been related to changes in chondrocyte morphology, further suggesting a complex system of regulatory pathways coordinating biomechanical, metabolic, and morphologic properties of chondrocytes.[23]

UNIQUE PROPERTIES OF ANKLE CARTILAGE IN COMPARISON TO KNEE CARTILAGE
Chondrocytes: Differences Between Ankle and Knee

It has been proposed that inherent differences between ankle and knee chondrocytes may provide ankles with greater resistance than knees to injury and subsequent development of OA.[17,45] One difference is that there is a greater density of chondrocytes in ankle cartilage than in knee cartilage.[17] Increased cellularity in cartilage may amplify cartilage's metabolic ability for repair by increasing the cumulative capacity of chondrocytes to reverse imbalances between anabolism and catabolism.[17]

Ankle cartilage may also be more tolerant to injury because it is less responsive than knee cartilage to catabolic stimuli that promote cartilage degeneration.[45] This is supported by reports that explant cultures of knee cartilage are up to eight times more responsive to IL-1 stimulation of PG synthesis suppression than ankle cartilage explants.[45,64] The increased sensitivity of knee cartilage to catabolic stimuli is not limited to cytokine signaling but includes catabolic pathways regulated though ECM interactions with chondrocytes.[46] This is supported by in vitro studies showing greater catabolic response of knee cartilage to the damaging effects of Fnfs.[64] Fnfs are one of the most potent and extensively studied matrix degradation products known to promote cartilage degeneration.[9,46]

Differences in chondrocyte sensitivity to matrix and cytokine responses within and among joints may mean that the development of promising cytokine or matrix molecule–based therapies for OA in the knee may not be as effective in the ankle. In addition, cytokine-based therapies that principally act through effects on superficial chondrocyte activities would only be efficacious in early stages of OA rather than in later stages of OA, in which the superficial zone is no longer intact. These nuances may be critical considerations in future strategies for cytokine-based therapies for the treatment of OA that may be focused toward joint-specific or stage-specific intervention.

Matrix: Differences Between Ankle and Knee

Ankle cartilage has a higher PG content and basal rate of PG synthesis than knee cartilage.[17,65] Ankle cartilage also has a lower water content than knee cartilage.[66] Biochemical differences between ankle and knee cartilage largely account for differences in biomechanical properties of cartilage from these joints. Ankle cartilage has a higher equilibrium modulus, greater dynamic stiffness, and lower hydraulic permeability than knee cartilage.[65] These properties may provide ankle cartilage with greater resistance to mechanical injury than knee cartilage.[65,66]

In studies comparing matrix turnover in normal and early-stage OA in ankles and knees, distinct differences were noted in how cartilage from each of these joints responded to injury. Comparisons of normal and degenerated ankles showed up-regulation of markers for collagen and PG synthesis.[41] These findings suggest that ankle cartilage responds to early injury by increasing anabolism with attempts at cartilage

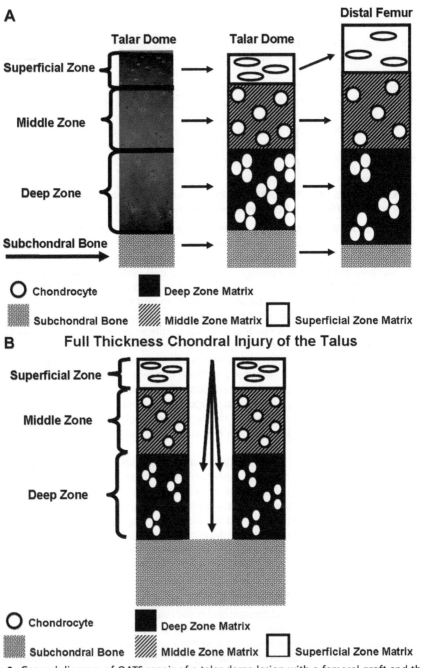

Fig. 2. General diagram of OATS repair of a talar dome lesion with a femoral graft and the potential sites of metabolic stress raiser formation. (*A*) General histology diagram compares talus and knee cartilage. The diagram highlights similar organization of cartilage by zones but gross differences in cartilage thickness between ankle and knee cartilage. (*B*) General diagram of a full-thickness defect in cartilage before repair with a femoral osteochondral transplant. (*C*) General diagram of a cartilage defect after femoral osteochondral transplantation. Note the potential metabolic stress raisers in areas of malalignment of cartilage zones between the femoral graft and talus. Note the gross difference in cartilage thickness between the femur and talus that accounts for malalignment of zones.

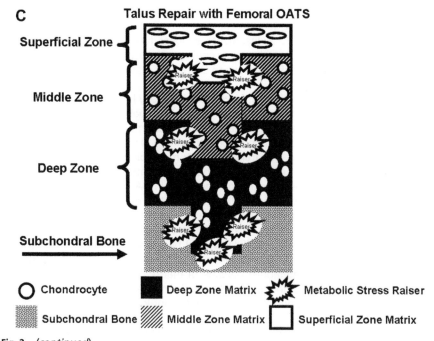

Fig. 2. (*continued*)

repair.[41] These same markers were shown to be down-regulated when comparing normal and degenerated knees.[41] These findings suggest that the early ankle cartilage response to degenerative processes is to rebuild matrix. It is not clear why knee cartilage does not display a similar increase in anabolism. It is interesting to speculate that an early attempt of knee cartilage to increase anabolism may be suppressed by early accumulation of matrix degradation products that do not accumulate in ankle cartilage because of its increased stiffness.[41,66]

Morphology: Differences Between Ankle and Knee

Comparative morphologic studies of knee and ankle chondrocytes show differences in spatial arrangements of superficial zone chondrocytes between ankles and knees.[67] Categoric comparison of uniaxial and biaxial joints demonstrates a distinct association between chondrocyte organization and joint dynamics.[67] Uniaxial joints, such as the ankle, have chondrocytes predominantly arranged in pairs, whereas knee chondrocytes are predominantly organized in strings.[67] It is not clear whether spatial arrangements are a result of sheer forces on chondrocyte morphology or have an essential function in cartilage homeostasis. Further understanding of spatial arrangements of chondrocytes may assist in the development of cartilage implants that are specific for joints and the location of injury.[67]

BRIDGING ADVANCEMENTS IN SCIENCE WITH LIMITATIONS IN CLINICAL CARE
Autologous Osteochondral Transplantation: Scientific Challenges and Limitations

Autologous osteochondral transplantation (OATS) is a procedure used in treatment of focal chondral injuries.[68–70] The procedure involves procurement and transplantation of full-thickness osteochondral grafts to regions of injury. Grafts are harvested from a non–weight-bearing region of the distal femur or from allogenic talus.[68–70] Few data are available regarding the long-term clinical and biologic success of OATS, although early clinical and arthroscopic assessments suggest functional improvement and gross incorporation of the grafts with hyaline cartilage-like properties.[70] Despite promising results, there are potential limitations to OATS that may challenge the long-term success of this treatment.[70]

Stress raisers are concentrations of force that potentially lead to mechanical failure of materials. Stress raisers commonly occur at junctions between two surfaces or at material interfaces with different mechanical and deformation properties. Classic cartilage failure from a stress raiser could be attributable to physical wear and fatigue, such as fibrillation or fissuring. In cartilage, matrix metabolism reciprocally regulates the mechanical properties of cartilage. Disturbances in matrix metabolism potentially alter the mechanical properties of cartilage and result in OA. Likewise, a disruption in joint mechanics can alter matrix metabolism and result in cartilage degeneration.

Metabolic stress raisers occur when there is an unnatural disruption in the continuity of two apposing matrix surfaces. Metabolic stress raisers may be caused by differences in matrix composition, cellularity, and basal matrix metabolism between two apposing tissues. These stress raisers potentially limit integration of graft and host by compromising the metabolic balance of matrix anabolism and catabolism. Without uniform integration of the graft and host, the native shock-absorbing properties of cartilage are lost, in addition to appropriate joint-loading forces that promote cartilage health.

A metabolic stress raiser potentially occurs at OATS sites when the cartilaginous zones of a graft and host are not symmetrically aligned (**Fig. 2**). Metabolic stress raisers occur by two means: (1) placement of an orthotopic talus graft proud or oversunk in relation to the host articular surface and (2) use of a femoral osteochondral graft to repair a talar lesion. Placement of a femoral graft into the talus may represent the most significant source of a metabolic stress raiser because of the mismatch in cartilage thicknesses, zone alignments, mechanical properties, matrix compositions, and matrix organization (see **Fig. 2**). Talus cartilage thickness is approximately 1.5 mm.[71] The cartilage thickness of the distal femur is between 2 and 6 mm, with the greatest thickness in the intercondylar regions.[71,72] Mismatched apposition of cartilage zones of a graft and host likely results in subtle alterations in matrix-to-matrix and cell-to-matrix interactions at the graft-host interface. These alterations potentially result in aberrant mechanical, biochemical, and matrix-related signaling that potentially disrupts the long-term metabolic equilibrium and long-term health of cartilage. These sites are metabolic stress raisers (see **Fig. 2**). The long-term presence of fibrocartilage at OATS-graft interfaces potentially represents a metabolic stress raiser and failure to maintain cartilage homeostasis, because fibrocartilage represents a form of scar tissue with inferior properties to native hyaline cartilage. Further research is necessary to clarify the significance and long-term implications of potential metabolic stress raisers. The phenomenon of metabolic stress raisers may also be pertinent to tissue engineering strategies, in which tissue regeneration constructs possess modulus and physical properties resembling native tissues but ultimately fail over time because of late effects of metabolic stress raisers between the construct and host.

The subchondral bone is also a site of stress raiser formation with osteochondral grafting. Increased subchondral stiffness during graft healing is a likely cause of increased load at the graft-host interface that results in stress raiser formation. Stress raisers have been demonstrated in goat models of OATS procedures, in which biomechanical analysis of OATS sites showed increased mechanical stiffness.[73] Increased stiffness was associated with increased trabecular mass in regions of healing subchondral bone.[73] Although no gross evidence of joint degeneration was noted, stress raisers at the subchondral graft interface may ultimately compromise the long-term loading dynamics of cartilage that are vital for maintaining cartilage homeostasis and health. A recent study correlating the angulation of subchondral trabecular bone orientation to regions of cartilage damage further supports how subchondral bone changes related to bone healing or native differences between knee and ankle cartilage may compromise the long-term health of cartilage after OATS.[74] Autogenous and allogenic grafts may be prone to subchondral stress raiser formation. Subchondral stress raisers most likely occur regardless of the autogenic or allogenic nature of grafting.

Despite these potential shortcomings in long-term durability of OATS techniques, longer term results by Hangody and colleagues[70] report good clinical and histologic appearances after treatment. Further studies and comparison of allogenic and autogenous grafts should be helpful in evaluating the likelihood and significance of mechanical and metabolic stress raisers in the long-term durability of OATs.

Autologous Chondrocyte Transplantation: Scientific Challenges and Limitations

Autologous chondrocyte transplantation (ACT) is a technique used in the treatment of focal chondral injuries.[75] With ACT, autogenous cartilage is taken from the knee and then enzymatically treated to release chondrocytes from the cartilage matrix

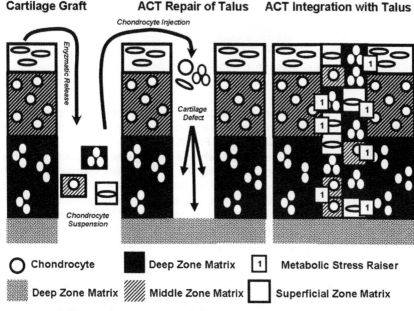

Fig. 3. General diagram for ACT repair of the talar dome and potential sites of metabolic stress raiser formation. A cartilage transplant is harvested from the knee, and chondrocytes are enzymatically released from the cartilage matrix. Chondrocytes are then replicated in tissue culture. Chondrocytes are next placed in suspension and injected into the cartilage defect. Transplanted chondrocytes then attempt repair and integration with talus cartilage. Because chondrocytes in suspension lack the native regulatory signals from ECM, they may not be able to reorganize effectively into the appropriate zones necessary to recapitulate structure and function. Superficial, deep, and middle zone chondrocytes may inappropriately repopulate zones in which they normally do not function. This may result in inappropriate interactions among cells and matrix components, resulting in metabolic stress raiser formation.

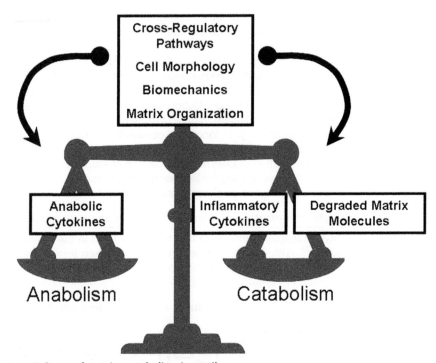

Fig. 4. Balance of matrix metabolism in cartilage.

(**Figs. 3** and **4**). Chondrocytes are then propagated in tissue culture. Propagated cells are released from culture and transplanted to a focal lesion in the talus after debridement and preparation of the host site (see **Fig. 3**).[76]

A significant concern of ACT is how and where a heterogeneous population of chondrocytes in suspension get the biologic signals to reorganize themselves into the appropriate zones with proper morphology, spatial organization, and density to recapitulate native cartilage structure, function, and metabolism. In native cartilage, the ECM provides many of the signals, and disruption of the ECM clearly results in cartilage degeneration as previously described. It is not clear whether in vivo cells in suspension use alternate signaling pathways than their matrix-bound counterparts or nonspecific signaling when the native extracellular environment is not available to guide metabolism and function. Matrix-deficient organization of chondrocytes may result in cartilage repair without restoring zone organization. Chondrocytes that are naturally present in the superficial zone have the opportunity to populate deeper layers of the regenerate layer, and deep zone cells may repopulate superficial layers (see **Fig. 3**). A heterogeneous population of chondrocytes throughout the regenerate may result in multiple regions of metabolic stress raisers. Failure to restore organization of cartilage zones may result in a failure to restore the metabolic balance of cartilage that maintains cartilage health. It is interesting to speculate whether fibrocartilage within the ACT represents a metabolic imbalance or satellite collections of metabolic stress raisers.[76]

New generations of ACT have utilized scaffolds to deliver cells. Most of these approaches have used homogeneous scaffolds. A current limitation of homogeneous matrix scaffolds is that they potentially compromise long-term cartilage homeostasis with omission of minor matrix components and their unique properties. CaReS, a collagen scaffold produced by Fidia Advanced Biomaterials (Padua, Italy), is an example of a homogeneous three-dimensional scaffold used in clinical practice to deliver chondrocytes to injured cartilage.[77] Upcoming generations of cell transplantation techniques will likely explore layered scaffolds with cell seeding prior to transplantation. Cartilink-2 is a type I/type II bilayer collagen scaffold currently in clinical use for autologous chondrocyte transplantation (ACT) treatment of chondral injury. The author is not aware of any studies characterizing the regenerates from these two products or how they compare with ACT without scaffold systems.

REFERENCES

1. Buckwalter JA, Saltzman C, Brown T. The impact of osteoarthritis: implications for research. Clin Orthop Relat Res 2004;(Suppl 427):S6–15.
2. Praemer AfS, Rice DP. Musculoskeletal conditions in the United States. Rosemont (IL): American Academy of Orthopedic Surgeons; 1999;79.
3. Jackson DW, Simon TM, Aberman HM. Symptomatic articular cartilage degeneration: the impact in the new millennium. Clin Orthop Relat Res 2001;(Suppl 391): S14–25.
4. Felson DT, et al. The prevalence of knee osteoarthritis in the elderly. The Framingham Osteoarthritis Study. Arthritis Rheum 1987;30(8):914–8.
5. Saltzman CL, et al. Impact of comorbidities on the measurement of health in patients with ankle osteoarthritis. J Bone Joint Surg Am 2006;88(11): 2366–72.
6. Muddu AK, et al. Resolving fibrosis in the diseased liver: translating the scientific promise to the clinic. Int J Biochem Cell Biol 2007;39(4):695–714.
7. Lagente V, et al. Role of matrix metalloproteinases in the development of airway inflammation and remodeling. Braz J Med Biol Res 2005;38(10):1521–30.
8. Gadek JE, et al. Role of connective tissue proteases in the pathogenesis of chronic inflammatory lung disease. Environ Health Perspect 1984;55:297–306.
9. Homandberg GA. Potential regulation of cartilage metabolism in osteoarthritis by fibronectin fragments. Front Biosci 1999;4:D713–30.
10. Weber KT, et al. Collagen network of the myocardium: function, structural remodeling and regulatory mechanisms. J Mol Cell Cardiol 1994;26(3):279–92.
11. Poole AR, et al. Changes in cartilage metabolism in arthritis are reflected by altered serum and synovial fluid levels of the cartilage proteoglycan aggrecan. Implications for pathogenesis. J Clin Invest 1994;94(1):25–33.
12. Anthony Ratcliffe, Mow Van C. In: Comper WD, editor. 1st edition, Extracellular matrix, vol. 1. Canada: Harwood Academic Publisher; 1996. p. 1–476.
13. Kuettner KE. Biochemistry of articular cartilage in health and disease. Clin Biochem 1992;25(3):155–63.
14. Poole AR, et al. Composition and structure of articular cartilage: a template for tissue repair. Clin Orthop Relat Res 2001;(Suppl 391):S26–33.
15. Aydelotte MB, Kuettner KE. Differences between sub-populations of cultured bovine articular chondrocytes. I. Morphology and cartilage matrix production. Connect Tissue Res 1988;18(3):205–22.
16. Ratcliffe A, Fryer PR, Hardingham TE. The distribution of aggregating proteoglycans in articular cartilage: comparison of quantitative immunoelectron microscopy with radioimmunoassay and biochemical analysis. J Histochem Cytochem 1984;32(2):193–201.

17. Huch K. Knee and ankle: human joints with different susceptibility to osteoarthritis reveal different cartilage cellularity and matrix synthesis in vitro. Arch Orthop Trauma Surg 2001;121(6):301–6.
18. Muller FJ, et al. Centrifugal characterization of proteoglycans from various depth layers and weight-bearing areas of normal and abnormal human articular cartilage. J Orthop Res 1989;7(3):326–34.
19. Akizuki S, et al. Tensile properties of human knee joint cartilage: I. Influence of ionic conditions, weight bearing, and fibrillation on the tensile modulus. J Orthop Res 1986;4(4):379–92.
20. Broom ND, Marra DL. New structural concepts of articular cartilage demonstrated with a physical model. Connect Tissue Res 1985;14(1):1–8.
21. Rieppo J, et al. Structure-function relationships in enzymatically modified articular cartilage. Cells Tissues Organs 2003;175(3):121–32.
22. Lane Smith R, et al. Effects of shear stress on articular chondrocyte metabolism. Biorheology 2000;37(1–2):95–107.
23. Smith RL, et al. Effects of fluid-induced shear on articular chondrocyte morphology and metabolism in vitro. J Orthop Res 1995;13(6):824–31.
24. Su JL, et al. Detection of superficial zone protein in human and animal body fluids by cross-species monoclonal antibodies specific to superficial zone protein. Hybridoma 2001;20(3):149–57.
25. Schumacher BL, et al. A novel proteoglycan synthesized and secreted by chondrocytes of the superficial zone of articular cartilage. Arch Biochem Biophys 1994;311(1):144–52.
26. Flannery CR, et al. Articular cartilage superficial zone protein (SZP) is homologous to megakaryocyte stimulating factor precursor and is a multifunctional proteoglycan with potential growth-promoting, cytoprotective, and lubricating properties in cartilage metabolism. Biochem Biophys Res Commun 1999; 254(3):535–41.
27. Warman ML. Human genetic insights into skeletal development, growth, and homeostasis. Clin Orthop Relat Res 2000;(Suppl 379):S40–54.
28. Brodkin KR, Garcia AJ, Levenston ME. Chondrocyte phenotypes on different extracellular matrix monolayers. Biomaterials 2004;25(28):5929–38.
29. Youn I, et al. Zonal variations in the three-dimensional morphology of the chondron measured in situ using confocal microscopy. Osteoarthr Cartil 2006;14(9): 889–97.
30. Hauselmann HJ, et al. The superficial layer of human articular cartilage is more susceptible to interleukin-1-induced damage than the deeper layers. Arthritis Rheum 1996;39(3):478–88.
31. Pelletier JP, et al. Are cytokines involved in osteoarthritic pathophysiology? Semin Arthritis Rheum 1991;20(6 Suppl 2):12–25.
32. Aydelotte MB, et al. Influence of interleukin-1 on the morphology and proteoglycan metabolism of cultured bovine articular chondrocytes. Connect Tissue Res 1992;28(1–2):143–59.
33. Salter DM, et al. Integrin-interleukin-4 mechanotransduction pathways in human chondrocytes. Clin Orthop Relat Res 2001;(Suppl 391):S49–60.
34. Scully SP, et al. The role of the extracellular matrix in articular chondrocyte regulation. Clin Orthop Relat Res 2001;(Suppl 391):S72–89.
35. Loeser RF. Integrin-mediated attachment of articular chondrocytes to extracellular matrix proteins. Arthritis Rheum 1993;36(8):1103–10.
36. Benton HP, Tyler JA. Inhibition of cartilage proteoglycan synthesis by interleukin I. Biochem Biophys Res Commun 1988;154(1):421–8.

37. Shinmei M, et al. Production of cytokines by chondrocytes and its role in proteoglycan degradation. J Rheumatol Suppl 1991;27:89–91.
38. Lee HS, et al. Integrin and mechanosensitive ion channel-dependent tyrosine phosphorylation of focal adhesion proteins and beta-catenin in human articular chondrocytes after mechanical stimulation. J Bone Miner Res 2000;15(8): 1501–9.
39. Chowdhury TT, et al. Dynamic compression counteracts IL-1beta induced inducible nitric oxide synthase and cyclo-oxygenase-2 expression in chondrocyte/ agarose constructs. Arthritis Res Ther 2008;10(2):R35.
40. Chubinskaya S, et al. Synergistic effect of IGF-1 and OP-1 on matrix formation by normal and OA chondrocytes cultured in alginate beads. Osteoarthr Cartil 2007; 15(4):421–30.
41. Aurich M, et al. Matrix homeostasis in aging normal human ankle cartilage. Arthritis Rheum 2002;46(11):2903–10.
42. Roughley PJ, Mort JS. Ageing and the aggregating proteoglycans of human articular cartilage. Clin Sci (Lond) 1986;71(4):337–44.
43. Bayliss MT, Ali SY. Age-related changes in the composition and structure of human articular-cartilage proteoglycans. Biochem J 1978;176(3):683–93.
44. Glant TT, et al. Age-related changes in protein-related epitopes of human articular-cartilage proteoglycans. Biochem J 1986;236(1):71–5.
45. Cole AA, Kuettner KE. Molecular basis for differences between human joints. Cell Mol Life Sci 2002;59(1):19–26.
46. Homandberg GA. Cartilage damage by matrix degradation products: fibronectin fragments. Clin Orthop Relat Res 2001;(Suppl 391):S100–7.
47. Jennings L, et al. The effects of collagen fragments on the extracellular matrix metabolism of bovine and human chondrocytes. Connect Tissue Res 2001; 42(1):71–86.
48. Knudson W, et al. Hyaluronan oligosaccharides perturb cartilage matrix homeostasis and induce chondrocytic chondrolysis. Arthritis Rheum 2000;43(5): 1165–74.
49. Grodzinsky AJ, et al. Cartilage tissue remodeling in response to mechanical forces. Annu Rev Biomed Eng 2000;2:691–713.
50. Setton LA, et al. Mechanical properties of canine articular cartilage are significantly altered following transection of the anterior cruciate ligament. J Orthop Res 1994;12(4):451–63.
51. Beaupre GS, Stevens SS, Carter DR. Mechanobiology in the development, maintenance, and degeneration of articular cartilage. J Rehabil R D 2000;37(2): 145–51.
52. Ramsey PL, Hamilton W. Changes in tibiotalar area of contact caused by lateral talar shift. J Bone Joint Surg Am 1976;58(3):356–7.
53. Paley D. In: Herzenberg J, editor. Principles of deformity correction. 1st edition. New York: Springer; 2003. p. 806.
54. Klein TJ, et al. Depth-dependent biomechanical and biochemical properties of fetal, newborn, and tissue-engineered articular cartilage. J Biomech 2007; 40(1):182–90.
55. Chen AC, et al. Depth- and strain-dependent mechanical and electromechanical properties of full-thickness bovine articular cartilage in confined compression. J Biomech 2001;34(1):1–12.
56. Brama PA, et al. Functional adaptation of equine articular cartilage: the formation of regional biochemical characteristics up to age one year. Equine Vet J 2000; 32(3):217–21.

57. Little CB, Ghosh P. Variation in proteoglycan metabolism by articular chondrocytes in different joint regions is determined by post-natal mechanical loading. Osteoarthr Cartil 1997;5(1):49–62.
58. Mohtai M, et al. Expression of interleukin-6 in osteoarthritic chondrocytes and effects of fluid-induced shear on this expression in normal human chondrocytes in vitro. J Orthop Res 1996;14(1):67–73.
59. Korver TH, et al. Effects of loading on the synthesis of proteoglycans in different layers of anatomically intact articular cartilage in vitro. J Rheumatol 1992;19(6): 905–12.
60. van Kampen GP, Korver GH, van de Stadt RJ. Modulation of proteoglycan composition in cultured anatomically intact joint cartilage by cyclic loads of various magnitudes. Int J Tissue React 1994;16(4):171–9.
61. Thibault M, Poole AR, Buschmann MD. Cyclic compression of cartilage/bone explants in vitro leads to physical weakening, mechanical breakdown of collagen and release of matrix fragments. J Orthop Res 2002;20(6):1265–73.
62. Nugent-Derfus GE, et al. Continuous passive motion applied to whole joints stimulates chondrocyte biosynthesis of PRG4. Osteoarthr Cartil 2007;15(5):566–74.
63. Waldman SD, et al. Long-term intermittent shear deformation improves the quality of cartilaginous tissue formed in vitro. J Orthop Res 2003;21(4):590–6.
64. Dang Y, Cole AA, Homandberg GA. Comparison of the catabolic effects of fibronectin fragments in human knee and ankle cartilages. Osteoarthr Cartil 2003; 11(7):538–47.
65. Treppo S, et al. Comparison of biomechanical and biochemical properties of cartilage from human knee and ankle pairs. J Orthop Res 2000;18(5):739–48.
66. Cole AA, Margulis A, Kuettner KE. Distinguishing ankle and knee articular cartilage. Foot Ankle Clin 2003;8(2):305–16, x.
67. Rolauffs B, et al. Distinct horizontal patterns in the spatial organization of superficial zone chondrocytes of human joints. J Struct Biol 2008;162(2):335–44.
68. Hangody L, et al. Mosaicplasty for the treatment of articular cartilage defects: application in clinical practice. Orthopedics 1998;21(7):751–6.
69. Hangody L, et al. Autologous osteochondral mosaicplasty. Surgical technique. J Bone Joint Surg Am 2004;86-A(Suppl 1):65–72.
70. Hangody L, et al. Autologous osteochondral grafting—technique and long-term results. Injury 2008;39(Suppl 1):S32–9.
71. Shepherd DE, Seedhom BB. Thickness of human articular cartilage in joints of the lower limb. Ann Rheum Dis 1999;58(1):27–34.
72. Kuettner KE, Cole AA. Cartilage degeneration in different human joints. Osteoarthr Cartil 2005;13(2):93–103.
73. Lane JG, et al. A morphologic, biochemical, and biomechanical assessment of short-term effects of osteochondral autograft plug transfer in an animal model. Arthroscopy 2001;17(8):856–63.
74. Schiff A, et al. Trabecular angle of the human talus is associated with the level of cartilage degeneration. J Musculoskelet Neuronal Interact 2007;7(3):224–30.
75. Brittberg M. Autologous chondrocyte implantation—technique and long-term follow-up. Injury 2008;39(Suppl 1):S40–9.
76. Whittaker JP, et al. Early results of autologous chondrocyte implantation in the talus. J Bone Joint Surg Br 2005;87(2):179–83.
77. Husing B, BB, Gaisser Sibyylle. Human tissue engineered products—today's market and future prospects. Fraunhauefer Karlsruhe, Germany: Institute for Systems and Innovation Research; 2003. p. 129.

MRI Evaluation of Ankle Distraction: A Preliminary Report

Bradley M. Lamm, DPM[a,*], Monique Gourdine-Shaw, DPM[b,c]

KEYWORDS

- Ankle distraction • MRI • Ankle arthritis • Ankle preservation
- Joint distraction • Cartilage repair • External fixation

A growing number of patients are seeking alternative treatment options for ankle arthritis other than arthrodesis or total joint replacement. Many patients prefer to preserve their natural ankle joint and ankle movement. Although research into cartilage regeneration and repair is promising, it is preliminary; nevertheless, at the current time, ankle distraction offers viable clinical outcomes.

Joint distraction with external fixation is an alternative to arthrodesis or joint replacement. The technique of joint distraction uses the principle of ligamentotaxis to restore the normal joint space, afford less joint loading, and provide an environment in which the joint cartilage can recover. The first reported joint distractions of the knee and elbow were performed in 1975, and joint distraction of the ankle was performed in 1978.[1,2] Aldegheri and colleagues,[3] from Verona, Italy, coined the term *arthrodiatasis* in 1979 to describe joint distraction [*arthro* (joint), *dia* (through), and *tasis* (to stretch out)].

Indications for ankle joint distraction are congruent joint surface, pain, joint mobility, and moderate to severe arthritis. The indications may be stretched to include avascular necrosis of the talus. Good clinical outcomes of ankle joint distraction with external fixation have been reported to range from 70% to 78% (studies by Paley and colleagues in 2008[4] and by van Roermund and colleagues).[5–12] The rationale as to why joint distraction is successful is largely unknown. Therefore, the purpose of this study was to evaluate pre- and postoperative ankle MRI scans of patients who underwent hinged ankle joint distraction with external fixation so as to understand better the effects of distraction on the joint.

[a] Podiatry Section, International Center for Limb Lengthening, Rubin Institute for Advanced Orthopedics, Sinai Hospital of Baltimore, 2401 West Belvedere Avenue, Baltimore, MD 21215, USA
[b] Medical Service Corps., United States Navy, United States Naval Academy, Annapolis, MD 21402, USA
[c] Veterans Affairs Maryland Healthcare Center, Baltimore, MD 21201, USA
* Corresponding author.
E-mail address: blamm@lifebridgehealth.org (B.M. Lamm).

Clin Podiatr Med Surg 26 (2009) 185–191
doi:10.1016/j.cpm.2008.12.007
0891-8422/08/$ – see front matter
© 2009 Elsevier Inc. All rights reserved.
podiatric.theclinics.com

EXISTING METHOD AND RESULTS

van Roermund and his coworkers[5–12] have written at length about the treatment of arthritis of the ankle with joint distraction. Ankle distraction treatment removes the mechanical stress (weight-bearing forces) on the cartilage to allow for restoration. Weight bearing with the external fixator allows for continued intermittent intra-articular fluid pressure and increased synovial fluid, which further aids in cartilage restoration. Maintaining the fixator for 3 months allows for reduction in the subchondral bone density, which increases the resilience of the joint. These effects of joint distraction allow for cartilage repair (ie, fibrocartilage).

The protocol that the Dutch group uses involves application of the Ilizarov device (a two-ring construct) to the tibia with two 1.5-mm Kirschner wires per ring attached by means of four threaded rods to a U-shaped foot ring (closed distally). A talar wire to prevent distraction of the subtalar joint, two crossing calcaneal olive wires, and one medial olive wire through the metatarsals are fixed to the foot ring. Distraction is performed at a rate of 0.5 mm two times per day for 5 days to achieve a total distraction of 5 mm. This distraction is maintained for 3 months, during which full weight bearing is allowed. The device is not hinged.

van Roermund and his coworkers[5–12] report that 70% of their patients showed significant clinical improvement, including a decrease in pain and increase in function (results for 50 patients with 2–8 years of follow-up). Joint mobility was sustained with the distraction treatment but was markedly restricted (50% of normal range). Most notable was the timing of the clinical improvement, with only one half of the clinical improvement occurring within the first year after the procedure. A slight increase in joint mobility, significant widening of the joint space, and diminished subchondral sclerosis were progressively observed during the 5 years after the procedure. These researchers also performed a prospective controlled study showing that joint distraction led to a statistically significant better clinical outcome than did arthroscopic débridement of the ankle joint alone.[5,8,9] In summary, van Roermund and his colleagues[5,6] showed that static ankle distraction alone without range-of-motion exercises yields a positive clinical effect in 70% of cases.

BALTIMORE TECHNIQUE
Hinged Ankle Joint Distraction

Unlike the Dutch group, the authors prefer to build their ankle distractor with an anatomically located hinge, which allows the patient to perform range-of-motion exercises throughout the entire distraction treatment. Inman's axis of the ankle joint is located during surgery, and universal hinges are placed medial and lateral to allow for hinged motion about this axis during treatment.[13] In addition, the authors combine concomitant correction of osseous alignment, muscle and joint contractures, and joint impingement to improve results.

ADJUNCTIVE PROCEDURES
Blocking Osteophyte Resection

If dorsiflexion is limited by anterior distal tibial or talar neck osteophytes, the osteophytes should be resected. An anterior approach is used to resect the anterior distal tibia and to deepen the neck of the talus. If plantarflexion is limited by posterior ankle osteophytes, they should be resected through a posterolateral incision (ie, Gallie approach) to gain access to the posterior ankle capsule. To prevent recurrence of these osteophytes, bone wax may be pressed into the cancellous bone. The authors also use nonsteroidal anti-inflammatory drugs (NSAIDs) (eg, indomethacin, naproxen) after surgery to inhibit bone formation for 6 weeks. However, NSAIDs are not used if an osteotomy is performed concomitantly.[14]

Equinus Contracture Release

Isolated anterior or posterior gastrocnemius recession (Baumann or Strayer procedure, respectively), gastrocnemius-soleus recession (modified Vulpius procedure), or Achilles tendon lengthening can be performed to correct equinus contracture.[15–17] The authors prefer the isolated gastrocnemius recession or gastrocnemius-soleus recession to maintain triceps surae muscle strength. A posterior capsular release may also be required to restore the ankle joint motion if the aforementioned procedures are not enough to correct the equinus. Tarsal tunnel decompression should be considered in acute and gradual correction of equinus contractures.[18] The tarsal tunnel decompression and the posterior ankle capsular release can be accomplished through a posteromedial longitudinal incision. The posterior osteophytes can also be resected through a posteromedial incision. When acute release is not sufficient to reduce the equinus, the residual equinus can be corrected using gradual distraction.

Ankle Joint Realignment

Ankle joint malalignment attributable to deformities (eg, valgus/varus, recurvatum/procurvatum, internal/external rotation) may be the cause of ankle joint degeneration.[16] To increase the longevity of the ankle joint cartilage, reorientation procedures, such as supramalleolar osteotomy, realign the ankle joint plafond. Subtalar contractures can be acutely reduced through a release or gradually corrected with the use of an external fixator. It is important to assess compensatory deformities accurately before surgical intervention.[16,19] Correction of ankle alignment is usually done using a supramalleolar osteotomy. This can be carried out acutely and fixed internally while the distraction is performed with external fixation. An alternative is to perform acute or gradual distal tibial realignment and ankle distraction with the same external fixator.

Distraction of 2 mm is performed in the operating room to ensure symmetric ankle joint distraction. Then distraction starts at a rate of 1 mm per day on postoperative day 1 for a total of 5 days. The goal is to achieve 8 to 10 mm of symmetric ankle joint distraction. The external fixation device is maintained for 3 months while allowing weight bearing as tolerated. The patient removes the posterior distraction rod to perform daily ankle range-of-motion exercises and attends physical therapy three times a week during the distraction treatment.

MATERIALS AND METHODS

The authors retrospectively reviewed the charts of three patients (three ankles) who underwent hinged ankle distraction with external fixation and had a minimum of 1-year of follow-up. All patients were diagnosed with painful ankle arthrosis based on clinical and radiographic evidence, and all patients were offered ankle fusion as an alterative treatment. The senior author (BML) performed the operation on the aforementioned patients between 2005 and 2007. The following information was obtained from the patients' records: gender, age, follow-up time, method of distraction, length of distraction, and preoperative diagnosis.

Pre- and postoperative T1- and T2-weighted sagittal and coronal MRI scans were collected from all three patients. The average duration between the time of surgery and the follow-up MRI was calculated. On the pre- and postoperative MRI scans, the subchondral bone thickness on the tibia and talus, the cartilage thickness or joint space, and the number and size of the subchondral bone cysts were measured. Measurements were performed with a ruler with 0.5-mm increments.

RETROSPECTIVE REVIEW RESULTS

Three patients' (two men and one woman) pre- and postoperative MRI scans were available for review. The average age of the patients was 41 years. Two right ankles and one left ankle underwent hinged ankle joint distraction. The preoperative diagnoses were posttraumatic ankle arthritis in all three patients. The average duration of treatment with external fixation was 4 months, followed by 1 month in a walking cast.

The pre- and postoperative T1- and T2-weighted sagittal and coronal MRI scans were compared. The postoperative MRI scan was obtained an average of 13 months after the initial distraction surgery. The MRI comparisons showed that the average postoperative subchondral bone thickness decreased by 0.5 mm, the average postoperative cartilage thickness or joint space increased by an average of 0.5 mm, and the average subchondral bone cysts of the talus and tibia decreased in number and size.

As a case example, a 44-year-old man with posttraumatic ankle arthritis underwent removal of the anterior ankle osteophytes and hinged ankle joint distraction with an external fixator (**Figs. 1–4**). The fixator was sustained for 4 months and then removed. MRI scans were obtained before surgery and 12 months after surgery. Note that the MRI scan was taken 8 months after removal of external fixator.

DISCUSSION

The reason why ankle distraction leads to lasting pain relief when treating ankle joint osteoarthritis is still speculative. It is possible that distraction permits cartilage repair to occur in a protected low-pressure environment. Salter and colleagues[20] showed that cartilage repair (fibrocartilage) occurs within a cartilage defect. Similarly, fibrocartilage formation was seen on the postoperative MRI scans in the current study.

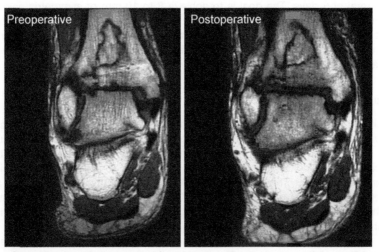

Fig. 1. Preoperative and postoperative T1-weighted coronal MRI scans. The ankle joint space or cartilage thickness is wider after surgery.

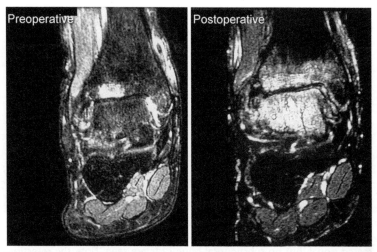

Fig. 2. Preoperative and postoperative T2-weighted coronal MRI scans. The subchondral bone cyst of the tibia has become diffuse. The tibia and talus have increased signal, but no subchondral bone cysts are seen.

Fibrocartilage formation is the body's attempt to restore a normal joint surface. Pain from osteoarthritis may be related to the effect of hydrostatic pressure on a subchondral bone cyst, whereby the synovial fluid from the joint enters through a cartilage defect (cavity) and increases the fluid, and thus the pressure, within the subchondral bone cyst.[10] Joint distraction allows for the formation of fibrocartilage, which adequately seals the cartilaginous cavity to the subchondral bone cyst, and therefore eliminates the increased fluid (pressure) and the pain.

Radiographs obtained after the external fixation is removed show that the joint distraction space of the ankle is not maintained. Typically, the radiographic joint space looks unchanged approximately 1 to 2 months after removal of external fixation.

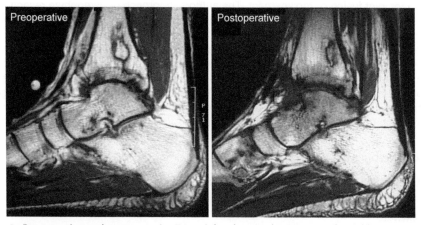

Fig. 3. Preoperative and postoperative T1-weighted sagittal MRI scans. The ankle joint space or cartilage thickness is wider after surgery. The subchondral bone thickness after surgery may have slightly decreased.

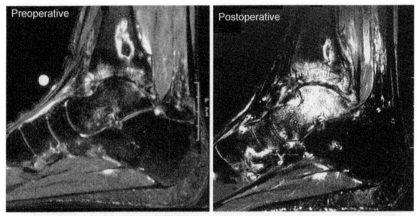

Fig. 4. Preoperative and postoperative T2-weighted sagittal MRI scans. The subchondral bone cysts of the tibia and talus have become diffuse after surgery. The tibia and talus have increased signal, but no subchondral bone cysts are seen. Note the resection of the anterior tibial osteophytes and the deepening of the talar neck.

Cartilage repair (ie, fibrocartilage) occurs during treatment, and the increased joint space or fibrocartilage after external fixation removal can be measured on the MRI scans. The findings of the MRI study show an increase of 0.5 mm of fibrocartilage, which has not been previously reported.

The authors' results showed decreased thickness of the subchondral bone after surgery. This finding has also been reported by the Dutch group in previous radiographic studies.[5–12] This response to the 4 months of ankle distraction is beneficial because it increases the resiliency of the cartilage overlying the subchondral bone.

SUMMARY

Ankle joint distraction is a viable alternative to ankle arthrodesis or ankle replacement. The main goal of ankle joint distraction is to decrease or eliminate pain and to delay the need for joint fusion or replacement. The authors' approach of osteophyte resection, muscle and joint contracture release, and osseous ankle realignment procedures, along with hinged ankle joint distraction, has proved to be clinically successful.[13] The reason(s) why joint distraction is successful is largely unknown. This preliminary pre- and postoperative MRI comparison study showed that fibrocartilage forms during the 4 months of joint distraction, increasing joint space (0.5 mm), which has not been reported in previous radiographic studies. Theoretically, the formation of fibrocartilage merely seals the cartilage cracks and eliminates the synovial filling of the subchondral bone cyst, thereby decreasing the joint pain.

ACKNOWLEDGMENTS

The authors thank Alvien Lee for his graphic design and photographic expertise.

REFERENCES

1. Volkov MV, Oganesian OV. Restoration of function in the knee and elbow with a hinge-distractor apparatus. J Bone Joint Surg Am 1975;57(5):591–600.

2. Judet R, Judet T. [The use of a hinge distraction apparatus after arthrolysis and arthroplasty]. Rev Chir Orthop Reparatrice Appar Mot 1978;64(5):353–65 [in French].
3. Aldegheri R, Trivella G, Saleh M. Articulated distraction of the hip: conservative surgery for arthritis in young patients. Clin Orthop Relat Res 1994;301:94–101.
4. Paley D, Lamm BM, Purohit RM, et al. Distraction arthroplasty of the ankle–how far can you stretch the indications? Foot Ankle Clin 2008;13:471–84.
5. van Roermund PM, Marijnissen AC, Lafeber FP. Joint distraction as an alternative for the treatment of osteoarthritis. Foot Ankle Clin 2002;7(3):515–27.
6. Marijnissen AC, van Roermund PM, van Melkebeek J, et al. Clinical benefit of joint distraction in the treatment of ankle osteoarthritis. Foot Ankle Clin 2003;8(2): 335–46.
7. van Valburg AA, van Roermund PM, Marijnissen AC, et al. Joint distraction in treatment of osteoarthritis: a two-year follow-up of the ankle. Osteoarthr Cartil 1999;7(5):474–9.
8. Marijnissen AC, van Roermund PM, van Melkebeek J, et al. Clinical benefit of joint distraction in treatment of severe osteoarthritis of the ankle: proof of concept in an open prospective study and in a randomized controlled study. Arthritis Rheum 2002;46(11):2893–902.
9. Marijnissen AC, Vincken KL, Viergever MA, et al. Ankle images digital analysis (AIDA): digital measurement of joint space width and subchondral sclerosis on standard radiographs. Osteoarthr Cartil 2001;9(3):264–72.
10. Marijnissen AC, van Roermund PM, Verzijl N, et al. Does joint distraction result in actual repair of cartilage in experimentally induced osteoarthritis? Arthritis Rheum 2001;44:S306.
11. van Roermund PM, Lafeber FP. Joint distraction as treatment for ankle osteoarthritis. Instr Course Lect 1999;48:249–54.
12. van Valburg AA, van Roermund PM, Lammens J, et al. Can Ilizarov joint distraction delay the need for an arthrodesis of the ankle? A preliminary report. J Bone Joint Surg Br 1995;77(5):720–5.
13. Paley D, Lamm BM. Ankle joint distraction. Foot Ankle Clin 2005;10:685–98.
14. Dahners LE, Mullis BH. Effects of nonsteroidal anti-inflammatory drugs on bone formation and soft-tissue healing. J Am Acad Orthop Surg 2004;12(3):139–43.
15. Lamm BM, Paley D, Herzenberg JE. Gastrocnemius soleus recession: a simpler more limited approach. J Am Podiatr Med Assoc 2005;95(1):18–25.
16. Paley D. Principles of deformity correction. corrected 3rd printing. Revised edition. 1st edition. Berlin: Springer-Verlag; 2005.
17. Herzenberg JE, Lamm BM, Corwin C, et al. Isolated recession of the gastrocnemius muscle: the Baumann procedure. Foot Ankle Int 2007;28(11):1154–9.
18. Lamm BM, Paley D, Testani M, et al. Tarsal tunnel decompression in leg lengthening and deformity correction of the foot and ankle. J Foot Ankle Surg 2007; 46(3):201–6.
19. Lamm BM, Paley D. Deformity correction planning for hindfoot, ankle, and lower limb. Clin Podiatr Med Surg 2004;21(3):305–26.
20. Salter RB, Simmonds DF, Malcolm BW, et al. The biological effect of continuous passive motion on the healing of full-thickness defects in articular cartilage: an experimental investigation in the rabbit. J Bone Joint Surg Am 1980;62(8): 1232–51.

Brace Management for Ankle Arthritis

Shine John, DPM*, Frank Bongiovanni, DPM, C. Ped

KEYWORDS

• Ankle arthritis • Bracing • Osteoarthritis • AFO

Isolated ankle arthritis, regardless of origin, can be a difficult condition to treat. Ankle arthritis is relatively rare, and, most often, it is posttraumatically induced, which includes cartilaginous injury and ligamentous insufficiency.[1] Ankle arthrodesis remains the surgical goal standard for management of ankle arthritis. As with all arthrodesis procedures, it is not without the potential for nonunions and complications.[2,3] Bracing can play a key role in patients who have degenerative disease of the ankle because it can prolong surgical intervention.

Although various noncustom and custom braces are available, not all are well-suited to address ankle joint arthritis specifically. Devices like walker boots and generic ankle braces may be useful in the short term but are cumbersome, inadequate, and not ideal for long-term use.

This article discusses a practical approach in describing the types of braces, fabrication details, and modifications necessary for the practitioner to be better equipped to prescribe and evaluate braces for ankle arthritis.

BRACING GOALS

The ankle joint axis lies close to the transverse and frontal planes; thus, principal motion occurs in the sagittal plane as dorsiflexion and plantarflexion. Movement within the joint, even minimal in severe arthritic cases, can elicit a great deal of pain and limitation with weight bearing and ambulation. As ankle arthritis and deformity worsen, increased forces are transmitted through the subtalar and talonavicular joints and result in degenerative change.[4] An effective brace should therefore function to control and limit sagittal plane motion within the ankle joint and should maintain the joint in neutral position. Because of the design of these braces, total triplanar motion within the hind foot can be limited as well.

The practical aspect of bracing goals is patience compliance with the brace. Aspects like bulkiness, discomfort, and accessibility with shoe gear are factors that can contribute to patient apprehension. Understanding the fabrication, materials, and modifications is important in achieving success with patient satisfaction and compliance.

Weil Foot and Ankle Institute, 1455 Golf Road, Des Plaines, IL 60016, USA
* Corresponding author.
E-mail address: sj@weil4feet.com (S. John).

Clin Podiatr Med Surg 26 (2009) 193–197
doi:10.1016/j.cpm.2008.12.004
0891-8422/08/$ – see front matter © 2009 Elsevier Inc. All rights reserved.

podiatric.theclinics.com

BRACE MATERIALS AND SPECIFICATIONS

The most important concept in understanding brace technique is having an understanding of the plastic shell. The plastic shell (encompassed by two layers of leather) is the foundation of the brace. Creating a proper shell is more an art than a science. The concept is to maintain control (rigidity) in the malleoli area while creating flexibility in the distal portion of the brace corresponding to the plantar aspect of the foot. You accomplish this by beginning with a 0.125-inch polypropylene shell (thicker plastics create a bulky brace that compromises shoe fit). The plantar portion is to be grinded to 0.0625 inch, tapering proximally to 0.125 inch in the malleoli region. Bony prominences (most commonly, navicular tuberosity) need to be accommodated with 0.125-inch extra firm material (soft rubber). A plastic interface on bony prominences leads to pain and intolerance by patients. There should be no plastic in the heel portion, which is referred to as "hammocking the heel" (**Fig. 1**). This characteristic allows for easy shoe fit, prevents the need for split shoe sizes, and ensures less irritation at the patient's heel. The trim line of the distal shell should end at the midshaft of the first metatarsal on the medial aspect and at the base of the fifth metatarsal on the lateral side. This design allows for easy fit and usability. The standard height of these braces is 5 inches above the malleoli. Those patients who are older or exhibit skin atrophy can usually only tolerate braces 1 inch above the ankle. Patients who have a large distal leg girth with severe ankle pathologic findings usually require braces higher than 5 inches on the leg. Caution should be exercised with braces crafted higher than 5 inches, however, because they create a painful area in the posterior aspect of the leg. The plastic shell should be lined with 0.125-inch pink plastazote to provide a shock absorptive interface (**Fig. 2**). Poron has a tendency to create a bulky brace.

Leather selection is an important factor in brace fabrication. The senior author (F.B.) prefers garment leather because it is soft, thin, and moldable. Calfskin does wear

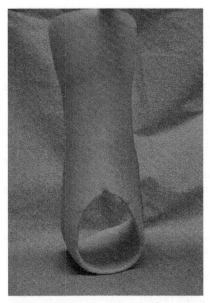

Fig. 1. "Hammocking" involves creating an opening in the posterior inferior distal portion within the inner plastic shell of the custom brace.

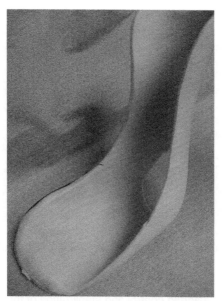

Fig. 2. The inner plastic shell is lined with 0.125-inch plastazote.

better but is harder and bulkier. Interior leather should be a natural tone (white or beige). This ensures that no dyes were used in the tanning process, which decreases heat production and the likelihood of an allergic reaction. Black exterior leather is the preferred color. Black leather, compared with other pigments, allows for necessary adjustments with a heat gun without destroying the cosmesis of the brace. It is important to remember that approximately 30% of braces require some type of adjustment to the plastic shell. Another important characteristic is that the interior leather not be glued to the plastic shell. To adjust the brace, one can pull the interior leather away from the plastic shell and apply heat to the black exterior leather. This allows the physician to transfer heat to the plastic shell, making it moldable. This design prevents destruction of the brace and makes adjustments fast and easy.

BRACE TYPES

The authors believe that custom ankle-foot orthosis (AFO) gauntlet braces are the "gold standard" for ankle and midfoot pathologic conditions (**Fig. 3**). Hinged AFO brace braces (ie, Richie brace) are nice in theory but create many pressure issues in the malleoli and navicular tuberosity area. There is no medial and lateral stability, which causes painful spots in the malleoli area. Another problem with these braces is the foot bed system, which does not allow accommodation of bony prominences with softer materials.

The carbon graphite AFO (ie, Allard ToeOff) is becoming popular in the treatment of degenerative joint disease and posterior tibial tendon dysfunction. The authors believe that this is erroneous. These braces should only be used for drop-foot deformities. Even with a custom foot bed system, they do not provide adequate frontal and transverse plane control.

In the presence of ankle arthritis combined with frontal plane deformity of the ankle, a custom brace on its own may be insufficient. In such cases, a custom AFO gauntlet may be used with a buttress shoe modification for added stability (**Fig. 4**). The

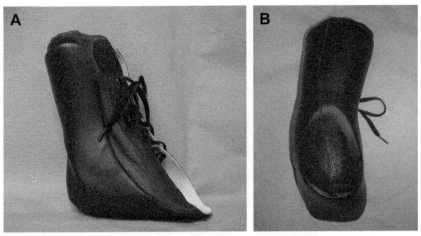

Fig. 3. (*A*) The finished custom gauntlet brace. (*B*) Final appearance of the brace with "hammocking" of the heel.

combination can provide added control and stabilization of the ankle when structural malalignment is present. Another useful modification is a rocker bottom sole, which can easily be incorporated into a patient's shoe (**Fig. 5**).

Extrinsic AFOs, such as double-upright braces, do provide adequate sagittal plane control but, unfortunately, may be inadequate in supplying frontal plane control. Devices like a patella weight-bearing device can offload and redistribute pressure

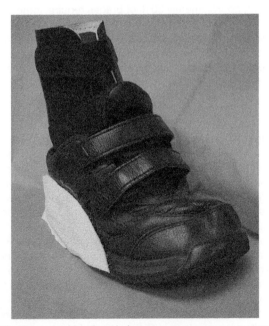

Fig. 4. Shoe modifications combined with brace management can accommodate frontal plane instability. A buttress can be added to the patient's shoe for added stability.

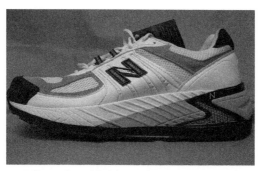

Fig. 5. A rocker bottom sole can be added to a patient's shoe or sneaker to assist in sagittal plane motion.

away from the hind foot. These devices can be combined with custom-made shoes in more advanced cases, such as those evidenced in patients who have rheumatoid arthritis. Many patients find these devices cosmetically displeasing and cumbersome, often leading to reduced patient compliance with the device.

SUMMARY

Management of ankle arthritis can be difficult for the physician and patient. Conservative options are limited but should be exhausted in an effort to prolong ankle arthrodesis. Custom braces can provide an effective means to alleviate pain, improve quality of life, and prolong ankle arthrodesis in patients affected by advanced ankle arthritis with or without deformity.

REFERENCES

1. Raikin SM. Arthrodesis of the ankle: arthroscopic, mini-open, and open techniques. Foot Ankle Clin 2003;8:347–59.
2. Frey C, Halikus NM, Vu-Rose T, et al. A review of ankle arthrodesis: predisposing factors to nonunion. Foot Ankle Int 1994;15:581–4.
3. Cooper PS. Complications of ankle and tibiotalocalcaneal arthrodesis. Clin Orthop Relat Res 2001;391:33–44.
4. Ahmad J, Raikin SM. Ankle arthrodesis: the simple and the complex. Foot Ankle Clin 2008 Sep;13(3):381–400.

Update on Viscosupplementation in the Treatment of Osteoarthritis of the Foot and Ankle

Kirk A. Grogan, DPM*, Thomas J. Chang, DPM, Robert S. Salk, DPM

KEYWORDS

- Viscosupplementation • Hyaluronans • Hyaluronic acid
- Osteoarthritis • Dejenerative joint disease • Synovial fluid
- Biosupplementation

The purpose of viscosupplementation in an osteoarthritic joint is to introduce hyaluronic acid (HA) into the joint to provide initial lubrication and shock absorption along with a long-term goal of changing the disease process of the joint.

HA is a high molecular weight polysaccharide and a major natural component of the synovial fluid and the extracellular matrix of the cartilage.[1] It is a glycosaminoglycan consisting of repeating units of glucuronic acid and N-acetylglucosamine, bound together by a glycoside bond beta. HA is synthesized by chondrocytes in the cartilage and fibroblasts of the synovial lining known as synoviocytes. The HA synthesized by the former becomes integrated in the cartilage matrix, whereas the synoviocyte HA is released in the synovial cavity. In degenerative joint diseases the average molecular weight and concentration of HA in the synovial fluid and the HA and proteoglycan content of the extracellular matrix of the cartilage is reduced. The rationale for use of HA is based on the concept of fluid replacement (viscosupplementation), and on the mounting evidence that HA plays a major role in biological activation (biosupplementation) that may decrease symptoms and disease progression.[1] The fact that all injected HAs are gone within days,[2] yet the clinical benefit lasts for months, suggests that biological activation is the dominant mechanism by which HAs mediate their clinical benefit.

PATHOLOGY OF OSTEOARTHRITIS

Osteoarthritis (OA) is a disease that may have different causes (eg, trauma, biomechanics) but similar biologic and clinical outcomes. The disease processes not only

Northern California Foot and Ankle Center
* Corresponding author.
E-mail address: kirk.grogan@gmail.com (K.A. Grogan).

Clin Podiatr Med Surg 26 (2009) 199–204
doi:10.1016/j.cpm.2009.03.001
0891-8422/09/$ – see front matter © 2009 Elsevier Inc. All rights reserved.

affect the articular cartilage but also involve the entire joint, including the subchondral bone, ligaments, capsule, synovial membrane, and periarticular muscles. Ultimately, the articular cartilage degenerates with fibrillation, fissures, ulceration, and full-thickness loss of the joint surface. OA is a result of both mechanical and biologic events that destabilize the normal coupling of degradation and synthesis of articular cartilage of chondrocytes and extracellular matrix, and subchondral bone. Ultimately, OA is manifested by morphologic, biochemical, molecular, and biomechanical changes of cells and matrix, which leads to a softening, fibrillation, ulceration, loss of articular cartilage, sclerosis, and eburnation of subchondral bone, osteophytes, and subchondral cysts. When clinically evident, OA is characterized by joint pain, tenderness, limitation of movement, crepitus, occasional effusion, and variable degrees of inflammation without systemic effects.[3]

In OA, the synovial fluid loses its elastic and viscous properties because of the changes in the molecular size and concentration of HA.[4] This change in physical properties results in a decrease in lubrication of the articulation and a lessening of shock absorption of the synovial fluid. HA is a shock absorber in the joint during fast movements and becomes a lubricant during slow movements. These qualities decrease in the arthritic joint, thus adding to the existing poor mechanics.

With respect to the ankle, arthritis is predictable after repeated soft tissue injuries or an intra-articular fracture. The incidence of ankle arthritis after ankle fracture is seen even after surgical anatomic reduction, yet anatomic repair may delay the onset because of restoration of optimal function and alignment. Patients are informed of this at the time of their initial injury and understand this is an unfortunate sequelae of their injury.

CHARACTERISTICS OF COMMERCIAL VISCOSUPPLEMENTS

There are currently five viscosupplements that are approved by the US Food and Drug Administration (FDA). These are Hyalgan, Supartz, Synvisc, Orthovisc, and Euflexxa. The HA in the first four is extracted from chicken combs. Euflexxa is bioengineered; therefore, any proteins that may cause reactions in some patients are absent.

The molecular weight of physiologic HA is 4 to 5 million daltons. In a diseased joint however, the molecular weight of the HA is reduced as the intrinsic HA starts to degrade. The molecular weight of the viscosupplements available in the United States range from 0.6 to 6 million daltons. Some studies show an advantage to using low-to-intermediate weight HA.[5] The weight (in millions of daltons) of the available viscosupplements is: Hyalgan 0.5 to 0.7, Supartz 0.6 to 1.2, Synvisc 6, Orthovisc 1 to 2.9, and Euflexxa 2.4 to 3.6. Synvisc contains 8 milligrams (mg) per milliliter (mL) of HA whereas Hyalgan, Supartz, and Euflexxa contain 10 mg per mL of HA. Orthovisc contains 15 mg per mL of HA.

Are all the hyaluronans created equal? Will all the injected materials produce the same clinical response? The half-life of all these products is only several days, yet the clinical response is often seen for much longer, sometimes up to one year. The efficacy of the injections is not just a consequence of lubrication and cushioning of the diseased joint. Smith and Ghosh[6] discussed the optimum molecular weight to facilitate the maximum amount of receptor binding. The receptor binding serves to provide the biologic activation of the joint and its synovial and chondrocyte receptors. This should equate to the maximum stimulation of intrinsic HA production, which seems to relate directly to the disease-modifying properties of these medications. As soon as the half-life wears off, it is important for the HA receptors inside the cell to be tightly bound. For optimum signal and binding, it is recommended that the hyaluronan be between .5 and 4 million daltons, whereas suboptimal binding seems to occur when the molecular weight is under .5 million daltons or over 4 million daltons. Therefore, it may be more likely for optimum binding to occur when using the lower molecular weight products. Synvisc possesses the highest viscosity and is possibly the best for joint cushioning, but that is only part of the picture.

Hyalgan and Supartz require five weekly injections, whereas Synvisc, Orthovisc, and Euflexxa require three weekly injections. The well-known clinical trial from Altman and Moskowitz,[7] which gained FDA approval for use of Hyalgan in the knee was performed with a five-injection protocol. Therefore, other investigators have also recommended five injections with the lower molecular weight (Hyalgan, Supartz) hyaluronans. Three injections have usually been reserved for the higher weight products.

PHYSIOLOGY OF VISCOSUPPLEMENTS

Besides the mechanical qualities of increasing viscosity and elasticity in the synovial fluid, HA injections produce several favorable physiological changes. They decrease inflammation within the joints.[8] They also increase the synthesis of endogenous HA by stimulating the production by the synovium. These qualities seem consistent with the fact that the HA placed within the joint is absent after a short period of time, but long-term clinical benefits are observed well after the product is gone.

Studies have also shown the disease-modifying benefits of viscosupplementation. The three parameters which have been well documented to show joint repair are: slowdown of joint space narrowing,[9] improvement in cartilage lesions from arthroscopic examination,[10,11] and improvement in structural features of the biopsied chondrocytes.[12] There is no placebo or injectable material which boasts these modifying benefits, and long-term cortisone injections have shown to be detrimental to cartilage viability.

RESEARCH ON HYALURONIC ACID USE IN THE FOOT AND ANKLE

There are few controlled trials involving the lower extremity. Salk and colleagues[13] used a double-blinded, placebo-controlled trial to show the efficacy of five weekly injections of HA (Hyalgan) in the ankle compared to normal saline. The patients were allowed to continue their activities of daily living with no assistive device. This study showed that the group receiving HA had a clinically significant decrease in pain compared to the placebo, which was phosphate-buffered saline. This study was the first well-designed, carefully controlled study to assess efficacy of HA for foot or ankle OA.

In addition to the therapeutic effects of hyaluronans before surgical treatment, there are studies that show its positive effects with perioperative and postoperative use.[14,15] Carpenter and Moxley[16] performed a study that showed that postoperative injections of HA (Synvisc) for 3 weeks after ankle arthroscopy was efficacious compared to ankle arthroscopy alone. The first injection was given 1 week after the arthroscopic procedure. The patients were allowed to be partially weight bearing with the use of crutches and a walking cast for the first week postoperatively, then fully weight bearing for the next 2 weeks. The walking cast was then discontinued after the third week.

Petrella and colleagues[17] performed a placebo-controlled study on acute lateral ankle sprains. In this study, they performed periarticular injections of either HA or saline on the day of and 4 days after the injury. Their study showed an overall decrease in pain and a quicker return to activity with HA.

Pons and colleagues[18] performed a study comparing the single injection of 1 mL of HA (Ostenil) into the first metatarsophalangeal joint with 1 mL of corticosteroid (triamcinolone acetonide) in the treatment of hallux rigidus. The patients in both arms of the study were to refrain from strenuous activity for a day after the injection. At 12-weeks follow-up, this single-blinded study showed a decrease in pain and an improvement in function in the HA group compared with the corticosteroid group. This study, conducted in Spain, did not involve a hyaluronate approved for use in the United States.

ADMINISTRATION OF VISCOSUPPLEMENTS

The administration of HA can be performed in the office without ultrasound or fluoroscopic guidance. Considering that the protocol requires at least three weekly injections (3 for Orthovisc, Euflexxa, and Synvisc; 5 for Supartz and Hyalgan), it may be helpful to alternate the injection site between the medial and lateral arthroscopic portals. The medial portal is medial to the tibialis anterior tendon and the lateral portal is lateral to the dorsal cutaneous nerve. An anterior central portal between the tibialis anterior and extensor hallucis longus tendon may also be helpful depending on the areas of damage.

At times, it is extremely difficult to find multiple portals of entry into an arthritic joint. Once an entry point is found for deep administration into the joint, it may be necessary to stay with the same approach throughout the treatment series. First, an aseptic prep is performed over the site. Next, a subcutaneous injection of local anesthetic is given to ease the placement of the larger gauge needle. The needle is inserted into the ankle joint and an aspiration is performed to make sure it is indeed within the joint. Then, all three mL of the HA is injected into the joint. The authors have also injected directly into the joint using a 25-gauge needle without a preinjection wheal, and have found the viscosity of the fluid easily travels through the needle without the need for a larger diameter. Fluoroscopic guidance may also be beneficial, but not necessary if there is careful clinical and radiographic evaluation before injection.

It may be more beneficial to use fluoroscopy when injecting into the subtalar joint. Because this imaging is often lacking at clinics, the posterolateral portal is a possible option for this joint. The patient is best placed in the prone or lateral position while the needle is inserted towards the subtalar joint between the peroneal tendons and the Achilles tendon at the level of the tip of the fibula. Another approach is into the anterior aspect of the posterior facet from the sinus tarsi.

The first metatarsophalangeal joint is injected using a dorsomedial and dorsolateral portal, with an option to alternate the approach each visit. The technique is the same as an injection of cortisone, which requires an angled approach that is proximal dorsal to distal plantar. This will help to avoid additional damage to the articular cartilage. It has the added benefit of allowing distraction of the hallux to aid placement.

The patient does not need to make transportation arrangements and can carry out their daily activities, with the exception of high impact activities such as running. The most common side effects of HA injections are pain, local swelling, and erythema around the injection site. Patients who are allergic to chicken or egg products should not use any HA except Euflexxa because of the risk of a reaction to the non-HA proteins.

At this time, the use of viscosupplementation in the foot and ankle is not FDA approved. Its' safety and efficacy has been demonstrated in Salk and colleagues' study and by anecdotal reports. It is to be hoped that these initial reports will stimulate companies' interest in pursuing further clinical trials and multicenter studies, and in seeking FDA approval. Currently, patients pay for the actual material used for each injection, although the patient visit and injection procedure is covered. The cost to the medical office of each vial is roughly $100 and adds up quickly when the recommended multiple injections are involved.

SUMMARY

In the recent past, nonsurgical treatment of OA was limited to rest, immobilization, physical therapy, activity modifications, nonsteroidal anti-inflammatory drugs, analgesics, weight loss, assistive devices for walking, and corticosteroid injections. The use of viscosupplementation is a welcome addition to the nonsurgical armamentarium that physicians have to treat OS. Additional studies are required, however, to test the safety and efficacy of this treatment in other parts of the foot.

REFERENCES

1. Swann DA. Macromolecules of synovial fluid. In: Sokoloff L, editor. The joints and synovial fluid. Orlando (FL): Academic Press; 1978. p. 407–35.
2. Abatangelo G, O'Regan M. Hyaluronan: biological role and function in articular joints. Eur J Rheumatol Inflamm 1995;15:492–501.
3. Brandt K, Dieppe P, Radin E. Etiopathogenesis of osteoarthritis. Rheum Dis Clin North Am 2008;34:531–59.
4. Fraser JR, Kimpton WG, Pierscionek BK, et al. The kinetics of hyaluronan in normal and acutely inflamed synovial joints: observations with experimental arthritis in sheep. Semin Arthritis Rhem 1993;22:9–17.
5. Vitanzo PC, Sennett BJ. Hyaluronans. Is clinical effectiveness dependent on molecular weight? Am J Orthop 2006;35:421–8.
6. Smith MM, Ghosh P. The synthesis of hyaluronic acid by human synovial fibroblasts is influenced by the nature of the hyaluronate in the extracellular environment. Rheumatol Int 1987;7:113–22.
7. Altman RD, Moskowitz R. Intraarticular sodium hyaluronate (Hyalgan) in the treatment of patients with osteoarthritis of the knee: a randomized clinical trial. J Rheumatol 1998;25:2203–12.
8. Punzi L, Schiavon F, Savasin F, et al. The influence of intra-articular hyaluronic acid on PGE2 and camp of synovial fluid. Clin Exp Rheumatol 1989;7:247–50.
9. Jubb RW, Piva S, Beinat L, et al. A one-year, randomised, placebo (saline) controlled clinical trial of 500-730 kDa sodium hyaluronate (Hyalgan) on the radiological change in osteoarthritis of the knee. Int J Clin Pract 2003;57(6):467–74.
10. Listrat V, Ayral X, Patarnello F, et al. Osteoarthritis and cartilage arthroscopic evaluation of potential structure modifying activity of hyaluronan (Hyalgan) in osteoarthritis of the knee. Osteoarthritis Cartilage 1997;5(3):153–60.
11. Frizziero L, Govoni E, Bacchini P. Intra-articular hyaluronic acid in the treatment of osteoarthritis of the knee: clinical and morphological study. Clin Exp Rheumatol 1998;16(4):441–9.
12. Guidolin DD, Ronchetti IP, Lini E, et al. Morphological analysis of articular cartilage biopsies from a randomized, clinical study comparing the effects of 500–730 kDa sodium hyaluronate (Hyalgan) and methylprednisolone acetate on primary osteoarthritis of the knee. Osteoarthritis Cartilage 2001;9(4):371–81.
13. Salk RS, Chang TJ, D'Costa W, et al. Sodium hyaluronate in the treatment of osteoarthritis of the ankle: a controlled, randomized, double-blinded pilot study. J Bone Joint Surg Am 2006;86A:295–302.

14. Wang CW, Gao LH, Jin XY, et al. The observation of the effectiveness of sodium hyaluronate injection after surgery. Chin J Reparative Reconstr Surg 2002;16(1): 1–8 [In Chinese].

15. Wang CW, Gao LH, Jin XY, et al. [Clinical study of sodium hyaluronate in supplementary treatment of comminuted fracture of ankle]. Chin J Reparative Reconstr Surg 2002;16(1):21–7 [In Chinese].

16. Carpenter B, Moxley T. The role of viscosupplementation in the ankle using Hylan G-F 20. J Foot Ankle Surg 2008;47:377–84.

17. Petrella RJ, Petrella MJ, Cogliano A. Periarticular hyaluronic acid in acute ankle sprain. Clin J Sport Med 2007;17(4):251–7.

18. Pons M, Alverez F, Solana J, et al. Sodium hyaluronate in the treatment of hallux rigidus. A single-blind, randomized study. Foot Ankle Int 2007;28:38–42.

A Review of Osteochondral Lesions of the Talus

Jordan P. Grossman, DPM, FACFAS*, Michael C. Lyons II, DPM

KEYWORDS

- Osteochondral lesion • OCD • OLT • Talar fracture
- Transchondral fracture • Ankle trauma

An osteochondral lesion of the talus (OLT) is defined as an injury to the talar dome that results in partial or total separation of the articular cartilage or subchondral bone. OLTs typically are preceded by a traumatic event and generally result in vascular damage to the subchondral bone. Many terms have been used for OLTs, such as osteochondral defects of the talus, talar dome lesions, osteochondral fracture, transchondral fracture, osteochondritis dissecans, and flake fractures.

Credit for originally describing OLTs of the ankle is given to Alexander Monro,[1] in his description in 1738. His initial observation was that they were loose osteocartilaginous bodies that were the result of trauma. The first description of any type of loose articular body and the subsequent removal from the knee is credited to Ambrose Pare,[2] in 1558. Paget,[3] in 1870, described a similar pathology in the patellofermoral joint, which was termed, *Paget's quiet necrosis of bone*.

The term, *osteochondritis dissecans*, was used later by Konig[4] in 1888, when he described loose bodies in other joints. He attributed these loose bodies to the result of spontaneous necrosis. In breaking down this nomenclature, the *-itis* implies inflammation, which has yet to be associated with the process. *Dissecans* is from the Latin root, *dissecare,* which means to separate. In 1922 Kappis[5] used osteochondritis dissecans to describe similar lesions in the ankle. Rendu,[6] in 1932, wrote of a case in which he discovered an intra-articular fracture of the talar dome that was identical to those reported by Kappis and Monro.

Berndt and Harty,[7] in 1959, devised the first classification of osteochondral lesions of the talus, still used to this day (**Box 1**). This study also helped to describe the mechanism by which these lesions occur. They coined the term, *transchondral fracture*.

The incidence of OLTs is only 0.09% of all fractures and 1% of talus fractures.[8] Of all osteochindritides, those involving the talus account for 4% of the total.[9] It is reported

---

Department of Orthopedics, Podiatry Section, St. Vincent Charity Hospital, 2351 E. 22nd Street, Cleveland, OH 44115, USA
* Corresponding author.
E-mail address: j.grossman@mac.com (J.P. Grossman).

Clin Podiatr Med Surg 26 (2009) 205–226
doi:10.1016/j.cpm.2009.01.003   podiatric.theclinics.com
0891-8422/09/$ – see front matter © 2009 Elsevier Inc. All rights reserved.

Box 1
Berndt–Harty staging

Stage I—Subchondral compression fracture

Stage II—Incomplete avulsion of fragment

Stage III—Compete avulsion of fragment without displacement

Stage IV—Complete avulsion with displacement

Data from Berndt AL, Harty M. Transchondral fractures (osteochondritis diseccans) of the talus. J Bone Joint Surg 1959;41A:988–1020.

---

that the prevalence is 0.002 per 1000 persons.[10] Because these lesions typically are undiagnosed, these numbers may be inordinately low.

Since Berndt and Harty's article, a plethora of literature has been written concerning case studies, mechanisms of injury, etiology, and treatments. This article aims to give an in-depth overview of the most current information available on osteochondral lesions of the talus.

ETIOLOGY

The primary noted and accepted cause of OLTs is trauma,[7,11–13] although others believe them to result from ischemia alone. In traumatic cases, 5% to 9% of ankle sprains result in osteochondral lesions.[14–16] Ankle fractures are associated with OLTs in a range of 28% to 73%.[17–20]

All theories include a role of ischemia, although not all include it as the primary cause. The related ischemia occurs to the subchondral bone typically in relation to a traumatic event. As the chondral fragment is devoid of blood supply, it slowly lyses from the underlying subchondral bone and may become an intra-articular fragment.

Genetics also plays a role in the development of OLTs.[21–24] A case report by Woods and Harris[24] showed that identical twins developed OLTs of the talus without traumatic etiology. Conway[25] proposed embolism of epiphyseal arteries, excessive brittleness of epiphyseal bone and low-grade infectious process as possible causes of OLTs. Bernstein[26] theorized that these lesions occur secondary to those predisposed to aseptic separation of articular osteocartilaginous fragments.

In regard to location of lesion, lateral lesions are caused by trauma 98% of the time. Medial lesions are associated with trauma up to 70% of the time.[8] The frequency seems to be 55% for medial lesions and 45% for lateral lesions.[7,27,28] It also is reported that 10% to 25% are bilateral.[7,29]

MECHANISM OF INJURY

In cadaveric models, Berndt and Harty[7] were able to reproduce OLTs through several deforming forces. By dorsiflexing the ankle and exerting an inversion force, they were able to produce lateral lesions. With a dorsiflexed ankle, the talus is in complete contact with the tibial plafond and both malleoli. When a strong inversion force is exerted, the talus is forced against the fibular articulation and can produce a stage I lesion. With continued force, the lesion eventually may detach or be sheared off the talar dome.

In the same study, the investigators were able to reproduce medial lesions by exerting an inversion force on a plantarflexed foot. With the foot in plantarflexion, the narrow aspect of the talar dome is within the ankle joint and the collateral ligaments are relaxed. With an inversion force, the posterior aspect of the medial axilla of the talus comes in direct contact with the tibia. With enough force, a stage I lesion may be produced. If there is external rotation of the tibia on the talus, the lesion eventually becomes detached or displaced into the joint.

The location of each lesion has its correlation with the mechanism. Lateral lesions typically are located on the anterior aspect of the talar dome, whereas medial lesions mostly are on the central to posterior aspect of the talar dome. The mechanisms described are typical of ankle sprains and fractures, explaining the high correlation of OLTs with both injuries.

CLINICAL PRESENTATION

Typically patients who have OLTs initially present with similar signs and symptoms of an ankle sprain. Usually they describe a history of injury or chronic instability. Patients complain of generalized ankle pain, swelling, and possible clicking or catching with ankle range of motion (ROM). In some instances ankle ROM is limited and painful. If a patient has a suspected ankle sprain but continues to complain of pain or limitations after 6 to 8 weeks of conservative care, there should be suspicion of an OLT.

On physical examination, palpation typically elicits pain at the anteromedial and anterolateral margins of the ankle joint. At times there may be pain with palpation of the posteromedial aspect of the joint. Absence of palpable pain, however, does not rule out an OLT. Dorsiflexion and plantarflexion of the ankle may be limited and reveal popping, clicking, or catching, which can signify an osteochondral or chondral lesion. There also may be an associated ankle effusion.

DIAGNOSTIC STUDIES

Historically, plain film radiographs were the study of choice for diagnosis of OLTs.[7] The use of plain films led to underdiagnosis of the OLTs. With the advancement of medical technology and imaging modalities, there are many more aids in diagnosing OLTs.

Plain Films

Radiographs are the first line of diagnosis. If visible on plain films, anterior and central OLTs may be seen as a radiopaque area at the talar shoulder (medial or lateral) with possibility of a detached portion of the bone (**Fig. 1**). Posterior lesions may be visualized by a mortise ankle view with a 4-cm heel rise, which is taken with the foot plantar flexed on the ankle.[30] It has been recorded that 30% to 43% of lesions may not be

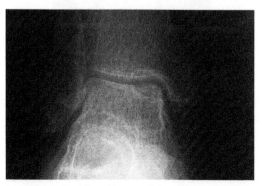

Fig. 1. Radiograph of medial OLT with evidence of detachment but not displacement.

visible on plain film radiographs.[8,30,31] The use of serial radiographs may reveal an OLT unseen on prior examination because a lesion progressed to a larger size (**Fig. 2**) or developed cystic changes. Other shortcomings are that the size and depth of lesions are unable to be determined and further investigation necessary.

Bone Scintigraphy

If radiographs are negative, but symptoms persist, scintigraphy may be used. Bone scintigraphy is useful in showing bony abnormalities by revealing changes in metabolism and blood flow to any area of bone.[32] Scintigraphy is useful as a screening method for detection of OLTs and generally not used for diagnosis. A retrospective study of 122 patients by Urman and colleagues[32] showed that scintigraphy has a sensitivity of 0.94 and specificity of 0.76. The investigators concluded that scintigraphy may give a relative location but is not valuable for determining the depth and size of lesions. If scintigraphy is negative, it helps to exclude OLT from the diagnosis and subsequently negate the need for further studies.[33]

MRI

MRI is the imaging study of choice for diagnosis of OLTs. It allows precise, noninvasive, nonradiating evaluation of location and extent of lesions (**Fig. 3**).[33,34] MRI has great soft tissue contrast, which allows for evaluation of cartilage, subchondral bone, cancellous bone, and synovium. It also allows for the relative determination of stability of lesions.[34,35] Lesion stability was characterized on MRI by Dipaola and colleagues[36] in 1991. They stated that stable lesions have intact overlying cartilage with solid fibrous or fibrocartilage attachment to underlying bone (**Fig. 4**). Unstable lesions have synovial fluid with granulation tissue between the fragment and crater (**Fig. 5**). MRI classifications have been described by Anderson and colleagues

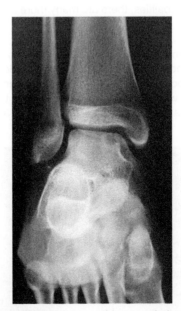

Fig. 2. Radiograph of large medial OLT. It is possible to track the size increase or decrease of larger lesions on plain film radiography.

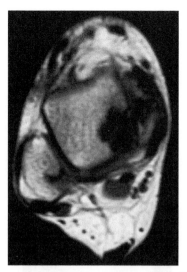

Fig. 3. MRI axial view of large medial OLT (the same patient as in **Fig. 2**).

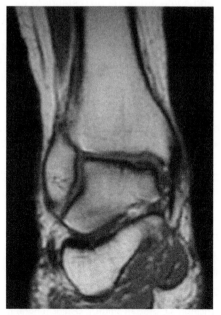

Fig. 4. MRI frontal view of medial OLT. Note the nondetachment but nondisplacement of the lesion.

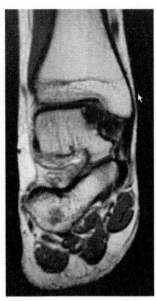

Fig. 5. MRI frontal view of large medial OLT (the same patient as in **Figs. 2** and **4**). Note the two large crater-like lesions.

(**Box 2**)[37] and Hepple and colleagues (**Box 3**).[31] Mintz and colleagues[38] have gone even further, classifying cartilage damage as depicted on MRI (**Box 4**).

CT

CT scans are valuable and some argue the gold standard for imaging OLTs.[33,39] CT scans, in the past, were the reference study for final diagnosis of OLTs.[32,33] Recently a CT classification has been proposed by Ferkel and coworkers (**Box 5**).[40] A study by Verhagen and colleagues[30] showed no statistical significance between CT and MRI for diagnosis of OLT. Although there is a high cost of CT scanning, it is valuable for preoperative planning in that it is best for identifying exact size and location of lesions.[39,41]

CONSERVATIVE THERAPY

With any pathology, conservative therapy should be exhausted before surgical intervention. Using the staging by Berndt and Harty, studies have shown that stage I

Box 2
MRI staging

Stage I—Subchondral compression fracture

Stage II—Incomplete separation of fragment

Stage IIa—Subchondral cyst formation

Stage III—Complete avulsion, nondisplaced

Stage IV—Displaced fragment

Data from Anderson IF, Crichton KJ, Grattan-Smith T. Osteochondral fractures of the dome of the talus. J Bone Joint Surg Am 1989;71(8):1143–52.

Box 3
MRI classification

Stage 1—Articular cartilage damage only

Stage 2a—Cartilage injury with fracture and bony edema

Stage 2b—Cartilage injury without bony edema

Stage 3—Detached, nondisplaced fragment

Stage 4—Detached and displaced fragment

Stage 5—Subchondral cyst formation

Data from Hepple S, Winson IG, Glew D. Osteochondral lesions of the talus: a revised classification. Foot Ankle Int 1999;20(12):789–93.

---

lesions should be treated with early protected ankle motion, consisting of taping, strapping, and ankle braces. Stage II lesions are treated with 4 to 6 weeks of immobilization, achieved with the use of short leg cast or controlled ankle motion walker/fracture boot. The efficacy of both treatment plans is 90%.[42] Canale and Belding used up to 18 weeks of immobilization for treatment of stage III lesions and found that medial lesions responded well to conservative therapy but lateral lesions necessitated operative intervention after failed conservative therapy.[29] The conclusion was made that stages I and II and medial III lesions can be treated conservatively, but lateral stage III and all stage IV lesions need surgical intervention.[29,42] Nonsteroidal anti-inflammatory drugs and cortisone injections may be used to decrease inflammation to the ankle joint. Physical therapy also may be instituted to aid in the healing of lesions.[7,29]

SURGICAL MANAGEMENT

Surgical intervention can be broken down into two categories, the first being surgical management without tissue transplantation and the other tissue transplantation. All the surgical options follow three general principles: débridement and bone marrow stimulation, fixation of talar dome lesion, and stimulation of hyaline cartilage formation. The authors of this article stratify surgical intervention into arthroscopy, arthrotomy, and malleolar osteotomy and details which techniques may be used with each exposure.

Once surgery is decided on, there are many factors that must be taken into consideration. Preoperatively, which surgical exposure and procedure are most ideal must

---

Box 4
MRI grading of talar dome cartilage

Grade 0—Normal cartilage

Grade 1—Abnormal signal, but intact

Grade 2—Fibrillation of fissures, not extending to bone

Grade 3—Flap present or bone exposed

Grade 4—Loose nondisplaced fragment

Grade 5—Displaced fragment

Data from Mintz DN, Tashjian GS, Connell DA, et al. Osteochondral lesions of the talus: a new magnetic resonance grading system with arthroscopic correlation. Arthroscopy 2003;19(4):353–9.

Box 5
CT classification

Stage I—Cystic lesion within talar dome, roof intact

Stage IIa—Cystic lesion with communication to talar dome

Stage IIb—Open articular surface lesion, nondisplaced fragment

Stage III—Nondisplaced lesion with lucency

Stage IV—Displaced fragment

Data from Ferkel RD, Sgaglione NA, Del Pizzo W. Arthroscopic treatment of osteochondral lesions of the talus: techniques and results. Orthop Trans 1990;14:172.

---

be decided. Certain factors are important, such as size of lesion, depth of lesion, type/stage of lesion, location of lesion, associated cystic changes, and viability of articular cartilage.

SURGICAL APPROACHES
Ankle Arthroscopy

Arthroscopy is described in the literature largely for the treatment of OLTs.[19,43–50] Techniques that may be used with arthroscopy include joint lavage and débridement, abrasion chondroplasty, subchondral drilling, and microfracture techniques. Lesions amenable to arthroscopy typically are those less than 1.5 cm.[51,52] OLTs with associated subchondral cystic involvement do poorly with arthroscopic management.[53] Many portal approaches are described, the most common including anteromedial, anterolateral, posterolateral, and transmalleolar.[54] There also are noninvasive ankle distractors that may be used to allow further visualization of the entire ankle joint.

The anterior portals are used most commonly (**Fig. 6**). For an anteromedial portal, the incision is longitudinal and just medial to the tibialis anterior tendon. The incision

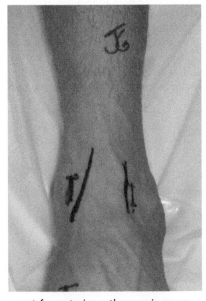

Fig. 6. Typical portal placement for anterior arthroscopic access.

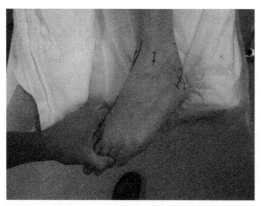

Fig. 7. This is the technique used to allow visualization of the Intermediate dorsal cutaneous nerve. The foot and fourth digit are maximally plantarflexed.

is approximately 5 mm in length and centered over the ankle joint. A curved hemostat is used to dilate the site and to identify the anterior ankle joint capsule. Introduction of the shaver or probe is into this portal. The anterolateral portal is, again, centered over the ankle joint, approximately 5 mm in length and is just lateral to the extensor tendons. The superficial peroneal nerve branch can be identified with simple plantarflexion of the foot and fourth digit (**Fig. 7**). This should make the nerve taut and easily visible cutaneously. This portal is similarly dilated and generally is the site for introduction of the arthroscope. With introduction of either instrument into the anterior portals, the foot must be dorsiflexed fully so as not to cause iatrogenic cartilaginous lesions (**Fig. 8**). The posterolateral portal is the safest of any posterior portal as it does not risk violation of the neurovascular bundle or the Achilles tendon. This portal generally is created after the scope has been inserted from an anterior portal. An 18-gauge spinal needle is placed just lateral to the Achilles tendon, then through the posterior capsule. Once it is visualized by the arthroscope, the needle is removed, a small stab incision made, and the obturator and trochar are inserted into the joint. The transmalleolar portal is used in association with drilling of the lesion. This portal typically is through the medial malleolus and small joint drill guide typically used.[54]

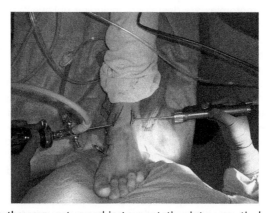

Fig. 8. Picture of arthroscopy setup and instrumentation intraoperatively.

Ankle Arthrotomy

Another surgical approach is via arthrotomy. This approach allows for good visualization of anterior lesions and generally is used for patients with lateral lesions. As described previously, most lateral lesions are located anteriorly, making them more amenable to simple arthrotomy. Because most medial lesions are central or posterior, they are harder to access with just ankle arthrotomy. Posterior arthrotomies are described,[55] although they are not used as commonly.

Anterolateral arthrotomies are performed most commonly.[55] The incision for this arthrotomy is an extension of the anterolateral portal. It is medial to the fibula and lateral to the extensor tendons and superficial peroneal nerve. The incision extends approximately 2 cm proximal and distal to the ankle joint. Once the incision is made, identification of the superficial peroneal nerve or its intermediate dorsal cutaneous branch is made and it is retracted. The extensor tendons are mobilized and retracted medially. At this point an incision is made into the ankle joint capsule. With simple plantarflexion and eversion, lateral lesions are accessible for treatment.

Anteromedial arthrotomies, although limited in their exposure, still are useful when accessing some medial lesions. The incision is made just medial to the tibialis anterior tendon and lateral to the great saphenous vein. This incision also extends 2 cm proximal and distal to the ankle joint. The tendon and vein are mobilized and retracted, giving view of the anteromedial aspect of the joint capsule. The capsule is then incised in line with the incision. This approach is not adequate for large medial lesions or lesions located more posteriorly.

The posterolateral approach also may be of use for gaining access to the ankle. This incision is placed posterior to the peroneal tendons at the level of the malleolus. Once through the subcutaneous tissue, the peroneal sheath and superior peroneal retinaculum are incised. The tendons are mobilized and retracted anteriorly. Any fatty tissue in the retrocalcaneal space needs to be retracted for full visualization of the ankle capsule. The capsule is incised and access to the posterolateral talus is achieved. This arthrotomy approach is used for posterolateral lesions or loose bodies and fragments.[55]

Malleolar Osteotomies

Malleolar osteotomies are described in several studies and include medial[8,12,28,50,56–62] or lateral[28,50,62–65] malleoli. Indications for malleolar osteotomy include posteromedial lesions, central lesions, and large medial and lateral lesions. Many orientations of medial malleolar osteotomies are described, including oblique,[61] transverse,[12] crescentic,[62] inverted V,[58] inverted U,[60] and step-cut.[59]

The authors' approach to medial malleolar osteotomy starts with incision just anterior to the midline of the tibia, starting approximately 4 cm proximal to the ankle joint and extending just distal to the tip of the malleolus. The incision may be biased slightly anterior to allow for adequate visualization of the anterior aspect of the tibia, proper osteotomy orientaton, and anatomic articular reduction. Dissection is performed through the subcutaneous tissue and the tibia identified. Care should be taken to identify and protect the greater saphenous vein and saphenous nerve. A small periosteal incision is made in line with the proposed osteotomy site. The tendon sheath of the tibialis posterior is incised and the tendon retracted posteriorly to prevent injury. If simple excision and subchondral drilling/microfracture are scheduled, an oblique osteotomy is performed, which is directed at the medial axilla of the tibial plafond. If an osteochondral transplantation procedure is anticipated, the orientation of the osteotomy should be more vertical to allow adequate visualization and instrument

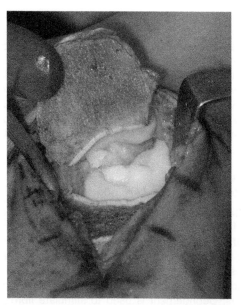

Fig. 9. Picture of the dorsomedial talus after medial malleolar osteotomy.

orientation to the talar dome. A sagittal saw is used to create the osteotomy but is not completed through the articular surface. Once the subchondral bone is encountered, the sagittal saw is removed and osteotome inserted to finish the cut. After completion of the cut, a sharp bone hook is used to retract the malleolar fragment inferiorly and visualization of the talar dome is achieved (**Fig. 9**). The deltoid ligaments are left intact.

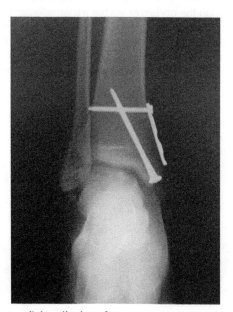

Fig. 10. Fixation of the medial malleolus after osteotomy. Note the two malleolar screws along with the 3-hole 1/3-in tubular plate with single screw fixation.

After completion of surgery, the malleolar fragment is reapproximated and fixated with screw fixation or, for the more vertically oriented osteotomies, an antiglide plate construct can be used. The plate generally is fixated with one screw in the proximal hole that is just superior to the osteotomy site (**Fig. 10**).

The approach to lateral malleolar osteotomy is a 5-cm incision placed just 1 cm proximal to tip of the malleolus and centered over the lateral midline of the fibula. Dissection is made down to bone with care not to transect any branches of the sural nerve. An oblique osteotomy is used to facilitate ease of fixation after the OLT is addressed. The authors prefer to use a 3.5-mm screw and a 1/3-in tubular neutralization plate for fixation.

SURGICAL TECHNIQUES
Débridement, Curettage, Drilling, and Microfracture

Débridement, curettage, drilling, or microfracture is used for stimulation of bone marrow. Violation of the subchondral bone results in formation of a fibrinous clot and a recruitment of mesenchymal stem cells. The result is filling in the lesion with fibrocartilage as the stem cells mature. This technique may be achieved with any of the three approaches described.

With the arthroscopic approach, débridement may be performed with abraders, shavers, and curettes. Débridement is used to stimulate fibrocartilage ingrowth. If any ankle synovitis or talotibial osteophytes are encountered, they can be débrided thoroughly with an arthroscopic blade, such as the Gator shaver or a full radius resector (ConMed Linvatec, Largo, Florida). Once all synovitis and osteophytes are débrided, a probe may be introduced and the foot plantarflexed as needed to palpate and identify the OLT. On visualization, a lesion may be débrided appropriately with a full radius resector or curetted with closed cup curette or ring curette and then the margins burred. It is of utmost importance that all unstable cartilage and any dead or devitalized subchondral bone be removed. Arthroscopic drilling and microfracture may be performed through the portals or via the transmalleolar portal.[39,53] Drilling and microfracture can be done by introduction of a microfracture probe, Steadman pick, Kirschner wire (K wire), or drill. The drill and K wire may be placed through the transmalleolar portal or through the anteromedial portal. If they are placed through the anteromedial portal, it is necessary to use a soft tissue sleeve to protect any vulnerable tissues.[50]

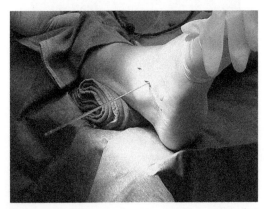

Fig. 11. View of needle insertion through the sinus tarsi as a guide for retrograde drilling. (*Courtesy of* Michael Lee, DPM, Des Moines, Iowa.)

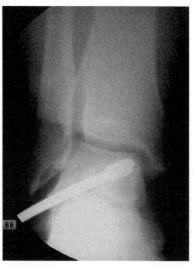

Fig.12. C-arm fluoroscopy of retrograde drilling. (*Courtesy of* Michael Lee, DPM, Des Moines, Iowa.)

In cases of subchondral cystic changes with intact viable cartilage, retrograde drilling also may be used. There are multiple intra-articular drill guides to aid in the ease of retrograde drilling. The guide is placed over the lesion and a K wire advanced through the sheath into the sinus tarsi and into the lesion, stopping just at the subchondral bone (**Fig. 11**). The technique commonly is used for medial lesions and is approached percutaneously through the sinus tarsi.[66] The area of the sinus tarsi that is drilled is the nonarticular junction of the head and neck. After insertion of the K wire, the intra-articular guide may be removed and drilling may commence (**Fig. 12**). Generally a 3.5-mm or 4.0-mm cannulated drill is used to drill into a lesion. The size of drill depends on lesion size. Drilling is performed under C-arm fluoroscopy with an anteroposterior ankle or mortise ankle view. Retrograde packing of the drill hole into the talar body and up to the subchondral bone then can be undertaken (**Fig. 13**). The bone graft

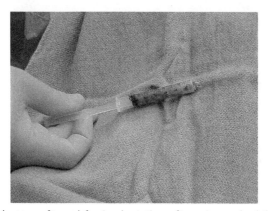

Fig. 13. Picture of bone graft used for implantation after retrograde drilling. (*Courtesy of* Michael Lee, DPM, Des Moines, Iowa.)

may be allograft or autograft. If autograft, the authors advocate the use of calcaneal bone graft or distal tibial bone graft.

Joint lavage, lesion excision, curettage, microfracture, and drilling are simple, effective ways to relieve mechanical symptoms.[50,53,66–69] A systematic review by Verhagen and colleagues[68] showed that excision alone had only a 38% success rate. Excision with curettage was successful in 76% of cases. Excision, curettage, and drilling had a success rate of 86%. Retrograde drilling alone had a success rate of 81% and, when combined with cancellous bone grafting, the success rate was up to 85%.

Osteochondral Transplantation

Osteochondral transplantation can be autologous, commonly from a patient's ipsilateral knee and[70–72] ipsilateral talus;[73,74] a fresh or frozen talar allograft; or synthetic products, such as OsteoCure Plug (Tornier, San Diego, California).

There are two basic types of osteochondral transplantation techniques: the osteochondral autograft transplant system (OATS) procedure and mosaicplasty. OATS is one osteochondral plug and a mosaicplasty uses multiple small grafts. A single graft, as in an OATS procedure, is considered better as there is a decrease in the fibrocartilage ingrowth. With mosaicplasty, fibrocartilage grows between each small graft. With the necessity of insertion of the grafts perpendicular to the recipient site, this type of procedure needs adequate exposure. For this reason, these lesions should be approached by arthrotomy or malleolar osteotomy. Typically, anterolateral lesions are accessible for implantation via arthrotomy and medial lesions via malleolar osteotomy. OATS and mosaicplasty are used for lesions greater than 10 mm in diameter.[71] If the choice is made to use a cadaveric talus, it is recommended to have magnification marked films taken so the proper sizing of the talus can be made. Once the proper size of talus is found, surgical intervention may proceed.

Prior to transplantation, the authors arthroscopically evaluate the ankle joint, débride any synovitis, and evaluate the lesion (**Fig. 14**). After arthroscopy, open access to the ankle is obtained (via the approach described previously). The lesion and any surrounding nonviable cartilage are débrided further (**Fig. 15**). Once the lesion is débrided and prepared fully, the mosaicplasty instruments or the OATS instruments

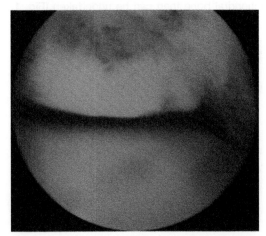

Fig. 14. Intraoperative arthroscopic view of the ankle joint after débridement of ankle synovitis.

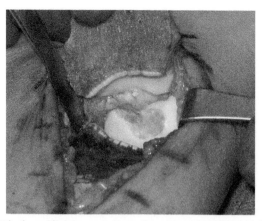

Fig. 15. View of OLT before débridement. Note the access via medial malleolar osteotomy.

are used to precisely measure the diameter and depth of the graft (**Fig. 16**). If mosaic-plasty is used, the necessary number of grafts can be determined. The talar recipient site is drilled for complete preparation (**Fig. 17**). For these procedures all the necessary instruments are in the manufacturer's set for preparation and implantation. Once the recipient site is prepared, the donor site is accessed. If autologous grafts are used, typically the lateral femoral condyle or the intercondylar femoral notch is the harvest site. Multiple grafts should be harvested for mosaicplasty or a single graft for OATS. Recommended depth is 25 mm,[50] and the graft should be at least twice the diameter needed. Procurement is by means of a double-edged tubular cutting chisel. Once the adequate graft or grafts are removed, a suction drain is placed in the knee and the area closed.

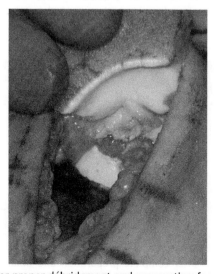

Fig. 16. View of OLT after proper débridement and preparation for autologous transfer.

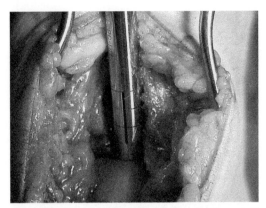

Fig. 17. Instrumentation used for drilling/measuring the depth and diameter of the OLT. (*Courtesy of* Michael Lee, DPM, Des Moines, Iowa.)

The ankle joint is revisited and flushed with normal saline. The delivery system from each set is used and the plug or plugs inserted. The same technique for delivery is used for the allograft implantation. All plugs are press fit and the ankle placed through a ROM to ensure there are no proud fragments and to aid in making the plugs more congruent (**Figs. 18** and **19**).

Open Reduction with Internal Fixation

Another strategy that may be used is fixation of a lesion, which may be performed with screws, pins, rods, or fibrin glue.[42,75,76] Malleolar osteotomy generally is required for fixation of any talar dome lesions, as simple arthrotomy does not offer enough access. Once the lesion is exposed, the choice of fixation is up to the surgeon. The authors have used TRIM-IT drill pins (Arthrex, Naples, Florida) and small headless screws for fixation and found easy handling and use of them. After fixation, the osteotomy is fixated (as described previously) and the patient placed in a modified Jones compression dressing with a posterior splint. The success rate of fixation is 73%.[68]

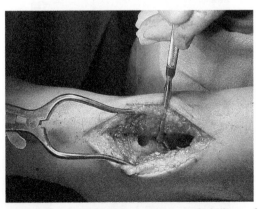

Fig. 18. View of the talus after complete preparation and drilling of the lesion before implantation (*Courtesy of* Michael Lee, DPM, Des Moines, Iowa.)

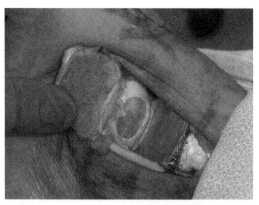

Fig. 19. View of talus after implantation of two allograft plugs.

Autologous Chondrocyte Implantation

First introduced in Sweden in 1987 for the knee, autologous chondrocyte implantation (ACI) is the implantation of in vitro cultured chondrocytes with the use of a periosteal tissue cover.[50,77] The use of ACI was brought into the mainstream by Brittberg and colleagues[78] with a success rate of 88% in the knee after 3-year follow-up. Since the use in knees, there have been reports of success in the talus.[77,79–82]

The technique begins with ankle arthroscopy, used to determine the size and depth of a lesion using a calibrated hook. A documentation form, as proposed by Petersen and colleagues,[81] may aid in the size determination of lesions. If there are any loose edges or loose bodies, they are removed. Once it is determined that ACI will be used, full-thickness slices of cartilage with a diameter of approximately 3 mm are removed from the femoral articular surface of the ipsilateral knee. Limited weight-bearing areas of the femur are used so as not to cause donor site morbidity. The slices are placed in a sterile container and sent to a bioengineering laboratory. The cartilage slices are cultured in the patient's own serum. The cultivation process takes approximately 2 to 3 weeks.[77]

Implantation access is with a malleolar osteotomy as this gives adequate exposure. Lesion site first is prepared via excision and curettage and removal of all loose fragments. A template is used to determine the defect size and pattern. A periosteal flap is dissected from the distal tibia for covering of the chondrocytes. The size and shape of the flap are determined by the template but 1 to 2 mm always are added to the size of the flap to ensure adequate coverage.[81] The periosteal flap is placed over the lesion with the cambrium layer down and sutured to the talar dome with 5-0 absorbable suture around the flap, leaving a small area open for implantation of the chondrocytes. Once ready, the chondrocytes should be injected with use of a flexible syringe and, after complete implantation, a final suture is placed. The malleolar osteotomy then is re-approximated (as described previously) and the patient placed in a modified Jones compression dressing with a posterior splint.

POSTOPERATIVE CARE

All patients are placed in a two-layer Jones compression dressing with a posterior splint. Patients who have undergone arthroscopy or arthrotomy with excision and curettage are immobilized for 2 weeks, then allowed to start ROM exercises at the 2-week mark. They are placed in a walking boot and are allowed weight bearing as

> **Box 6**
> **Treatment guidelines**
>
> *Lesion-Treatment*
>
> Type 1: asymptomatic or low-symptomatic lesions - Conservative
>
> Type 2: symptomatic lesion ≤10 mm - Débridement and drilling/microfracture
>
> Type 3: symptomatic lesion 11–14 mm - Débridement and drilling, fixation, osteochondral graft, or ACI
>
> Type 4: symptomatic lesion ≥15 mm - Fixation, graft, or ACI
>
> Type 5: large talar cyst - Retrograde drilling with or without bone transplant, or ACI
>
> Type 6: secondary lesion - Osteochondral transplant
>
> *Data from* Zengerink M, Szerb I, Hangody L, et al. Current concepts: treatment of osteochondral ankle defects. Foot Ankle Clin 2006;11:331–59.

tolerated. After the fourth week, they are started on physical therapy. At the 6-week mark patients may return to normal shoe gear and typically are given a lace-up ankle brace to ease the transition.

Patients who have undergone any procedure with malleolar osteotomy are kept non–weight bearing until radiographic healing is achieved, usually, approximately 6 to 8 weeks. At 2 weeks, patients are switched to a removable fracture boot. Non–weight-bearing home ROM exercises then are instituted. At approximately 6 weeks, physical therapy is instituted and patients may begin weight bearing once the osteotomy site is healed. Patients may transition to regular shoe gear at approximately the 10- to 12-week point. Again, a lace-up ankle brace is encouraged to help the transition.

SUMMARY

Most OLTs are the result of trauma and can be a cause of prolonged pain and disability. Investigation is warranted in patients who have ankle pain that is recalcitrant to normal therapies. There should be a low threshold for obtaining an MRI for further information. The authors recommend starting with an MRI if the diagnosis is unclear as it provides great detail for any possible soft tissue injury. If OLT is suspected or confirmed on radiograph, a CT may be ordered for best visualization of the size and depth.

As with all chronic conditions, conservative therapies must be exhausted first. If surgery is indicated, smaller lesions (<1.5 mm) without cystic changes are approached with arthroscopic débridement, curettage, and drilling. If a lesion is larger, other options should be instituted. The authors use autograft or synthetic osteochondral transplantation in lesions greater than 1.5 mm. The last resort is ACI and has great promise, although it is an expensive modality. Although there is not a widely accepted treatment guideline, Zengerink and colleagues have proposed a strategy (**Box 6**).

REFERENCES

1. Monro A. Part of the cartilage of the joint, separated and ossified. In: Medical essays and observations, vol. IV. Edinburgh (UK): Ruddinmans; 1738. p. 19.
2. Gross SD. A system of surgery: pathological, diagnostic, therapeutic, and operative. Volume 6. H.C. Lea's Son & Co.; 1882.

3. Paget J. On the production of the loose bodies in joints. St. Bartholomew's Hospital Reports 1870;6:1–4.
4. Konig F. Uber freie Korper in den gelenken. Deutsche Zeitschrift fur Chirurgie 1888;27:90–109 [In German].
5. Kappis M. Weitere beitrage zur traumatisch-mechanischen entstehung der "spontanen" knorpela biosungen. Deutsche Zeitschrift fur Chirurgie 1922;171: 13–29 [In German].
6. Rendu A. Fracture intra-articulair parcellaire de la poulie astragalienne. Lyon Med 1932;150:220–2 [In French].
7. Berndt AL, Harty M. Transchondral fractures (osteochondritis diseccans) of the talus. J Bone Joint Surg Am 1959;41A:988–1020.
8. Flick AB, Gould N. Osteochondritis dissecans of the talus (transchondral fractures of the talus): review of the literature and new surgical approach for medial dome lesions. Foot Ankle 1985;5(4):165–85.
9. Thompson JP, Loomer RL. Osteochondral lesions of the talus in a sports medicine clinic. A new radiographic technique and surgical approach. Am J Sports Med 1984;12(6):460–3.
10. Bauer M, Jonsson K, Linden B. Osteochondritis dissecans of the ankle. J Bone Joint Surg 1987;69-B(1):93–6.
11. Fairbank HAT. Osteochondritis dissecans. Br J Surg 1933;21:67–82.
12. Ray RB, Coughlin EJ. Osteochondritis dissecans. Beitr z Klin Chir 1932;150: 220–2.
13. Rödén S, Tillegárd P, Unander-Scharin L. Osteochondritis dissecans and similar lesions of the talus. Report of fifty-five cases with special reference to etiology and treatment. Acta Orthop Scand 1953;23:51–66.
14. Boisen WR, Staples OS, Russel SW. Residual disability following acute ankle sprains. J Bone Joint Surg Am 1955;37(6):1237–43.
15. Van Dijk CN. On diagnostic strategies in patients with severe ankle sprain (dissertation). Amsterdam the Netherlands: University of Amsterdam; 1994 [from Zengerink, et al].
16. Lippert MJ, Hawe W, Bernett P. Surgical therapy of fibular capsule-ligament rupture. Sportverletz Sportschaden 1989;3(1):6–13.
17. Sorrento DL, Mlodzienski A. Incidence of lateral talar dome lesions in SER IV ankle fractures. J Foot Ankle Surg 2000;39(6):354–7.
18. Hintermann B, Regazzoni P, Lampert C, et al. Arthroscopic findings in acute fractures of the ankle. J Bone Joint Surg Br 2000;82(3):345–51.
19. Takao M, Uchio Y, Naito K, et al. Diagnosis and treatment of combined intra-articular disorders in acute distal fibular fractures. J Trauma 2004;57(6): 1303–7.
20. Aktas S, Kocaoglu B, Gereli A, et al. Incidence of chondral lesions of talar dome in ankle fracture types. Foot Ankle Int 2008;29(3):287–92.
21. Wagoner G, Cohn BNE. Osteochondritis dissecans: a resume of the theories of etiology and the consideration of heredity as an etiologic factor. Arch Surg 1931;23:1–24.
22. Anderson DV, Lyne ED. Osteochondritis dissecans of the talus: case report on two family members. J Pediatr Orthop 1984;4(3):356–7.
23. Erban WK, Kolberg K. Simultaneous mirror image osteochondrosis dissecans in identical twins. Rofo 1981;135(3):357.
24. Woods K, Harris I. Osteochondritis dissecans of the talus in identical twins. J Bone Joint Surg Br 1995;77(2):331.

25. Conway FM. Osteochondritis dissecans. Intra-articular osseocartilaginous loose bodies. A clinical study based upon ten personally observed cases. Ann Surg 1934;99:410–31.

26. Bernstein MA. Osteochondritis dissecans. J Bone Joint Surg 1925;7:319–29.

27. McCullough CJ, Venugopal V. Osteochondritis dissecans of the talus: the natural history. Clin Orthop Relat Res 1979;144:264–8.

28. Davidson AM, Steele HD, MacKenzie DA, et al. A review of twenty-one cases of transchondral fracture of the talus. J Trauma 1967;7(3):378–415.

29. Canale ST, Belding RH. Osteochondral lesions of the talus. J Bone Joint Surg Am 1980;62(1):97–102.

30. Verhagen RA, Maas M, Dijkgraaf MG. Prospective study on diagnostic strategies in osteochondral lesions of the talus. Is MRI superior to helical CT? J Bone Joint Surg Br 2005;87(1):41–6.

31. Hepple S, Winson IG, Glew D. Osteochondral lesions of the talus: a revised classification. Foot Ankle Int 1999;20(12):789–93.

32. Urman M, Ammann W, Sisler J, et al. The role of bone scintigraphy in the evaluation of talar dome fractures. J Nucl Med 1991;32(12):2241–4.

33. Wells D, Oloff-Solomon J. Radiographic evaluation of transchondral dome fractures of the talus. J Foot Surg 1987;26:186–93.

34. Yulish BS, Mulopulos GP, Goodfellow DB, et al. MR imaging of osteochondral lesions of the talus. J Comput Assist Tomogr 1987;11:296–301.

35. DeSmet AA, Fisher DR, Burnstein MI, et al. Value of MR imaging in staging osteochondral lesions of the talus (osteochondritis dissecans). Am J Radiol 1985;154: 555–8.

36. Dipaola JD, Nelson DW, Colville MR. Characterizing osteochondral lesions by magnetic resonance imaging. Arthroscopy 1991;7:101–4.

37. Anderson IF, Crichton KJ, Grattan-Smith T. Osteochondral fractures of the dome of the talus. J Bone Joint Surg Am 1989;71(8):1143–52.

38. Mintz DN, Tashjian GS, Connell DA, et al. Osteochondral lesions of the talus: a new magnetic resonance grading system with arthroscopic correlation. Arthroscopy 2003;19(4):353–9.

39. Barnes CJ, Ferkel RD. Arthroscopic debridement and drilling of osteochondral lesions of the talus. Foot Ankle Clin 2003;8(2):243–57.

40. Ferkel RD, Sgaglione NA, Del Pizzo W. Arthroscopic treatment of osteochondral lesions of the talus: techniques and results. Orthop Trans 1990;14:172–8.

41. Lundeen RO, Stienstra JJ. Arthroscopic treatment of transchondral lesions of the talar dome. J Am Podiatr Med Assoc 1987;77(8):456–61.

42. Pettine KA, Morrey BF. Osteochondral fractures of the talus—a long-term follow-up. J Bone Joint Surg 1987;69B:89–92.

43. Baker CL, Andrews JR, Ryan JB. Arthroscopic treatment of transchondral talar dome fractures. Arthroscopy 1986;2(2):82–7.

44. Frank A, Cohen P, Beaufils P, et al. Arthroscopic treatment of osteochondral lesions of the talar dome. Arthroscopy 1989;5(1):57–61.

45. Kelberine F, Frank A. Arthroscopic treatment of osteochondral lesions of the talar dome: a retrospective study of 48 cases. Arthroscopy 1999;15(1):77–84.

46. Parisien JS. Arthroscopic treatment of osteochondral lesions of the talus. Am J Sports Med 1986;14(3):211–7.

47. Ferkel RD. Articular surface defects, loose bodies, and osteophytes. In: Arthroscopic surgery: the foot and ankle. Philadelphia: Lippincott-Raven; 1996. p. 145.

48. Tol JL, Struijs PA, Bossuyt PM, et al. Treatment strategies in osteochondral defects of the talar dome: a systematic review. Foot Ankle Int 2000;21(2):119–26.
49. Schuman L, Struijs PA, van Dijk CN. Arthroscopic treatment for osteochondral defects of the talus. Results at follow-up at 2 to 11 years. J Bone Joint Surg Br 2002;84(3):364–8.
50. Zengerink M, Szerb I, Hangody L, et al. Current concepts: treatment of osteochondral ankle defects. Foot Ankle Clin 2006;11:331–59.
51. Ogilvie-Harris DJ, Sarrosa EA. Arthroscopic treatment after previous failed open surgery for osteochondritis dissecans of the talus. Arthroscopy 1999;15(8):809–12.
52. Martin DF, Baker CL, Curl WW, et al. Operative ankle arthroscopy. Long term follow-up. Am J Sports Med 1989;17:16–23.
53. Kumai T, Takakura Y, Higashiyama I. Arthroscopic drilling for the treatment of osteochondral lesions of the talus. J Bone Joint Surg Am 1999;81(9):1229–35.
54. Ferkel RD, Scranton PE Jr. Arthroscopy of the ankle and foot. J Bone Joint Surg Am 1993;75(8):1233–42.
55. Navid DO, Myerson MS. Approach alternatives for treatment of osteochondral lesions of the talus. Foot Ankle Clin 2002;7:635–49.
56. Kelikian H, Kelikian AS. Osteocartilaginous bodies in and around the ankle joint. In: Kelikian H, Kelikian AS, editors. Disorders of the foot and ankle. Philadelphia: Saunders; 1985. p. 725–38.
57. Tachdjian MO. Acquired affections of bones, joints and soft tissues. In: Tachdjian MO, editor. The child's foot. Philadelphia: Saunders; 1985. p. 616–27.
58. O'Farrell TA, Costello BG. Osteochondritis dissecans of the talus. The late results of surgical treatment. J Bone Joint Surg 1982;64B:494–7.
59. Alexander IJ, Watson JT. Step-cut osteotomy of the medial malleolus for exposure of the medial ankle joint space. Foot Ankle 1991;11:242–3.
60. Oznur A. Medial malleolar window approach for osteochondral lesions of the talus. Foot Ankle Int 2001;22:841–2.
61. Spatt JF, Frank NG, Fox IM. Transchondral fractures of the dome of the talus. J Foot Surg 1986;25:68–72.
62. Wallen EA, Fallat LM. Crescentic transmalleolar osteotomy for optimal exposure of the medial talar dome. J foot Surg 1989;28:389–94.
63. Ly PN, Fallat LM. Transchondral fractures of the talus: a review of 64 surgical cases. J Foot Ankle Surg 1993;32:352–72.
64. Jakob RP, Mainil-Varlet P, Saage C, et al. Mosaicplasty in cartilaginous lesions over 4cm2 and indications outside the knee. Cartilage repair. Presented at the 2nd Fribourg International Symposium, Fribourg, Switzerland, October 29–31, 1997 (From Zengerink, et al).
65. Gautier E, Jung M, Mainil-Varlet P, et al. Articular surface repair in the talus using autogenous osteochondral plug transplantation. A preliminary report. Int Cartilage Rep Soc Newsletter 1999;1:19–20.
66. Taranow WS, Bisignani GA, Towers JD. Retrograde drilling of osteochondral lesions of the medial talar dome. Foot Ankle Int 1999;20(8):474–80.
67. van Dijk CN, Scholte D. Arthroscopy of the ankle joint. Arthroscopy 1997;13(1): 90–6.
68. Verhagen RA, Struijs PAA, Bossuyt PM, et al. Systematic review of treatment strategies for osteochondral defects of the talar dome. Foot Ankle Clin 2003;8(2): 233–42.
69. Thermann H, Becher C. Microfracture technique for treatment of osteochondral and degenerative chondral lesions of the talus. 2-year results of a prospective study. Unfallchirurgie 2004;107(1):27–32.

70. Hangody L, Kish G, Modis L. Mosaicplasty for the treatment of osteochondritis dissecans of the talus: two to seven year results in 36 patients. Foot Ankle Int 2001;22(7):552–8.

71. Hangody L, Kish G, Kárpáti Z, et al. Treatment of osteochondritis dissecans of the talus: use of the mosaicplasty technique—a preliminary report. Foot Ankle Int 1997;18(10):628–34.

72. Assenmacher JA, Kelikian AS, Gottlob C. Arthroscopically assisted autologous osteochondral transplantation for osteochondral lesions of the talar dome: an MRI and clinical follow-up study. Foot Ankle Int 2001;22(7):544–51.

73. Sammarco GJ, Makwana NK. Treatment of talar osteochondral lesions using local osteochondral graft. Foot Ankle Int 2002;23(8):693–8.

74. Kreuz PC, Steinwachs M, Erggelet C, et al. Mosaicplasty with autogenous talar autograft for osteochondral lesions of the talus after failed primary arthroscopic management: a prospective study with a 4-year follow-up. Am J Sports Med 2006;34(1):55–63.

75. Bruns J, Rosenbach B, Kahrs J. [Etiopathogenetic aspects of medial osteochondrosis dissecans tali]. Sportverletz Sportschaden 1992;6(2):43–9.

76. Zelent ME, Neese DJ. Talar dome fracture repaired using bioabsorbable fixation. J Am Podiatr Med Assoc 2006;96(3):256–9.

77. Baums MH, Heidrich G, Schultz W, et al. Autologous chondrocyte transplantation for treating cartilage defects of the talus. J Bone Joint Surg Am 2006;88(2):303–8.

78. Brittberg M, Lindahl A, Nilsson A. Treatment of deep cartilage defects in the knee with autologous chondrocyte transplantation. N Engl J Med 1994;331(14):889–95.

79. Giannini S, Vannini F, Buda R. Osteoarticular grafts in the treatment of OCD of the talus: mosaicplasty versus autologous chondrocyte transplantation. Foot Ankle Clin 2002;7(3):621–33.

80. Koulalis D, Schultz W, Heyden M. Autologous chondrocyte transplantation for osteochondritis dissecans of the talus. Clin Orthop 2002;(395):186–92.

81. Petersen L, Brittberg M, Lindahl A. Autologous chondrocyte transplantation of the ankle. Foot Ankle Clin 2003;8(2):291–303.

82. Whittaker JP, Smith G, Makwana N, et al. Early results of autologous chondrocyte implantation in the talus. J Bone Joint Surg Br 2005;87(2):179–83.

Ankle Arthrodiastasis

Andrew J. Kluesner, DPM[a], Dane K. Wukich, MD[b,c],*

KEYWORDS

- Ankle • Arthritis • Arthrodiastasis • Joint distraction
- Traumatic

Degenerative joint disease of the ankle remains a challenging problem for the foot and ankle surgeon. A recent multicenter study has concluded by objective evaluation that the mental and physical disability associated with end-stage ankle arthrosis is at least as severe as that associated with end-stage hip arthrosis.[1] Unlike the hip and knee joints, the ankle joint is rarely affected by primary osteoarthritis. Saltzman and colleagues[2] evaluated the cause of arthritis in a consecutive series of 639 arthritic ankles. The results demonstrated that 445 (70%) patients had posttraumatic arthritis, 76 (12%) had rheumatoid disease, and 46 (7%) had idiopathic arthritis (primary osteoarthritis).[2] As opposed to primary osteoarthritis, posttraumatic arthritis of the ankle joint presents a unique set of challenges because it generally occurs in a younger and more active population. Conservative treatment of ankle arthritis is primarily symptomatic in nature. When conservative treatment fails, surgical options include ankle joint arthrodesis, joint debridement, osteotomies, or joint replacement. Arthrodesis is considered the "gold standard" and has been shown to be effective at eliminating pain, but at the expense of loss of joint motion and overload of adjacent or contralateral joints. Recent long-term studies have reported increased disability associated with advancing arthrosis of adjacent joints after ankle arthrodesis.[3,4] The results of ankle joint replacements have been good; however, these implants have a limited lifespan and may not be indicated in the younger and more active patient. Ankle joint distraction, or arthrodiastasis, has been shown clinically to benefit patients significantly in the short-term and long-term treatment of ankle arthritis.[5] In a retrospective study of 22 patients 7 years after Ilizarov ankle joint distraction, 16 (73%) showed significant improvement in all clinical parameters studied.[6] Multiple

[a] Department of Surgery, University of Pittsburgh Medical Center, South Side Hospital, Pittsburgh, PA, USA
[b] Division of Foot and Ankle Surgery, Department of Orthopedic Surgery, University of Pittsburgh, Pittsburgh, PA, USA
[c] University of Pittsburgh Medical Center, Comprehensive Foot and Ankle Center, Roesch-Taylor Medical Building, 2100 Jane Street, Suite 7300, Pittsburgh, PA 15203, USA
* Corresponding author. University of Pittsburgh Medical Center, Comprehensive Foot and Ankle Center, Roesch-Taylor Medical Building, 2100 Jane Street, Suite 7300, Pittsburgh, PA 15203, USA
E-mail address: wukichdk@upmc.edu (D.K. Wukich).

Clin Podiatr Med Surg 26 (2009) 227–244
doi:10.1016/j.cpm.2008.12.006
0891-8422/08/$ – see front matter © 2009 Elsevier Inc. All rights reserved.

podiatric.theclinics.com

scientific studies have also demonstrated beneficial intra-articular changes with joint distraction.[7–10] For these reasons, arthrodiastasis, or ankle joint distraction, has emerged as a potential alternative treatment to decrease pain and improve joint function.

Ankle arthrodiastasis as a treatment for ankle arthritis is based on the theory that osteoarthritic cartilage in the ankle has healing capacity. A recent cadaveric study comparing cartilage in the knee joint with that in the ankle joint has suggested that ankle joint chondrocytes have a greater capacity for repair.[11] The reparative capacity of the chondrocyte is believed to be enhanced by mechanical offloading of the ankle joint by means of distraction with an external fixator, thus preventing further damage of the articular cartilage, unloading the periarticular bone, potentially decreasing the density of the subchondral bone, and allowing for decreased load on the overlying articular cartilage.[10] The chondrocyte repair is nourished by the maintenance of intra-articular fluid pressure changes within the joint. This intermittent flow is facilitated by joint movement with the use of hinges in the external fixator or by allowing the patient to walk with the frame in place. The flexibility of the frame, or motion with the hinges, allows intermittent increases in hydrostatic pressure, creating a supportive environment for cartilage repair.[10]

POSTTRAUMATIC ARTHRITIS

Articular cartilage provides elasticity and resistance to compressive forces, thus protecting the underlying bone. The properties of articular cartilage are conferred by the two major constituents of the cartilage extracellular matrix: collagens and proteoglycans. The chondrocyte is the functional cell of articular cartilage and is responsible for maintenance and production of the extracellular organic matrix. The normal adult chondrocyte, unless disturbed, remains in a quiescent state throughout life, exhibiting a decreased proliferative potential with age. Repetitive physiologic loading of the joint is vital to maintaining cartilage health. Intermittent intra-articular hydrostatic synovial fluid pressure changes are maintained by the normal cyclic loading of the joint associated with movement. These fluid pressure levels have been shown to inhibit cartilage degradation, angiogenesis, and ossification and to enhance the extracellular matrix.[12]

The development of osteoarthritis can be divided into two fundamental mechanisms related to the adverse affects of "abnormal" loading on normal cartilage or of "normal" loading on abnormal cartilage.[13] The first mechanism describes the most common posttraumatic cause of ankle joint arthritis (**Fig. 1**). Posttraumatic damage to the articular surfaces, ligaments, and capsule causes acute tissue injury, resulting in increased load transfer or altered patterns of load distribution that can accelerate the initiation and progression of osteoarthritis. Articular cartilage is particularly sensitive to pathologic changes in the loading rate, and there is evidence that increased loading rates may play a predominant role in the cause of posttraumatic osteoarthritis.[14]

Mechanical loading experiments on articular cartilage performed in vitro demonstrate that abnormal loading of the articular cartilage can significantly affect its composition, structure, metabolic activity, and mechanical properties.[15] Abnormal loading induces mechanical strain on the chondrocyte, causing an increase in oxidative stress. This oxidative stress is partially responsible for the age-related decline in cartilage health. As increased mechanical loading occurs, the oxidative stress on the chondrocyte also increases, potentially playing a role in accelerated cartilage senescence.[16] The effects of abnormal mechanical loading also contribute to dysregulation

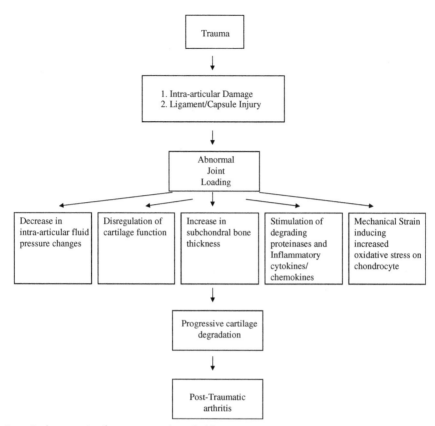

Fig. 1. Pathogenesis of posttraumatic arthritis.

of chondrocyte function, favoring disequilibrium between the catabolic and anabolic activities of the chondrocyte in remodeling the cartilage extracellular matrix. Chondrocytes have receptors for responding to mechanical stimulation that, when activated, stimulate the production of matrix-degrading proteinases and inflammatory cytokines and chemokines. Although not an inflammatory arthropathy, synovitis ensues secondarily with posttraumatic arthritis in response to cartilage breakdown products, further amplifying cartilage destruction. The cyclic intra-articular hydrostatic pressure has also been shown to be significantly lower in osteoarthritic joints, further affecting cartilage nutrition and breakdown.[12] Local loss of proteoglycans and cleavage of type II collagen occur initially at the cartilage surface, resulting in an increase in water content and loss of tensile strength in the cartilage as the disease progresses. In addition to the progressive loss of the articular cartilage, there is an increase in subchondral bone plate thickness, formation of new periarticular bone, subchondral sclerosis, and the development of subchondral cysts.[13]

Recently, attention has focused on the potential role of the subchondral bone in the development and progression of osteoarthritis. The development of cartilage degeneration is concomitant with increased subchondral bone thickness. The subchondral bone and deep cartilage layer act as a functional unit based on intricate canals connecting these two structures. Stiffer subchondral bone, caused by healed trabecular microfractures or the increased bony turnover seen in osteoarthritic bone, does not function as an effective shock absorber and may lead to articular cartilage damage. Additional evidence shows that vascular invasion and advancement in the zone of calcified cartilage from the tidemark region, at the junction of articular hyaline cartilage and subchondral bone, contribute to a decrease in the articular cartilage thickness. Structural alterations in the articular cartilage and periarticular bone caused by trauma may lead to alteration of the articular joint contours, further contributing to cartilage degeneration. A recent study also suggests that growth factors and cytokines derived directly from the subchondral bone may be responsible for the progression or initiation of osteoarthritis.[17] The relation between subchondral bone changes and the development of osteoarthritis continues to attract research interest.

HISTORICAL REVIEW

In 1975, Volkov and Oganesian[18] reported on the application of their hinged external fixation device to mobilize joint contractures, reduce old dislocations, and compress nonunited periarticular fractures of the elbow and knee. Once successful with these procedures, the external device was used to maintain separation of the joint surfaces, whereas the hinges allowed normal joint motion to be gradually restored. Encouraging results were reported in 31 knees and 28 elbows treated with this technique.[18] In 1978, Judet and Judet[19] first reported on joint distraction for osteoarthritis. These researchers created a cartilage layer defect in the joint surfaces of canine tibiotarsal joints and applied a hinged external fixator, maintaining 4 to 8 mm of joint space, for 30 days. Macroscopic and microscopic evaluation after the treatment period showed "callus with appearance close to that of normal articular cartilage." The use of monolateral hinged external fixators to stabilize and distract the elbow, knee, and ankle joints in patients who had osteoarthritis was also included in this study. A technique of articulated distraction combined with limited arthroplasty resulted in success for treatment of the elbow, knee, and ankle. "Good" results in 13 of the 16 ankles studied were reported at a follow-up time of 16 months.[19]

The term *arthrodiastasis* can be traced to Aldegheri,[20] who described a new regimen of articulated distraction and open surgery of the hip in 1979. The word was derived from the Greek *arthro* (joint), *dia* (through), and *tasis* (to stretch out). Aldegheri and colleagues[20] later reported on articulated joint distraction of the hip in a group of patients who had a variety of hip diseases, including osteoarthritis, ranging in age from 9 to 69 years. A hinged external fixator was used to maintain a joint space of 4 to 8 mm for 6 to 10 weeks. Satisfactory results were achieved in more than 70% (42 of 59) of the patients aged 45 years and younger; however, the procedure was ineffective in patients older than 45 years or with inflammatory arthropathy. These investigators concluded that articulated joint distraction was a viable treatment alternative in younger patients (<45 years of age). The results of these early studies stimulated interest in the study of joint distraction for ankle arthritis.

In 1995, van Valburg and colleagues[7] reported on a new approach for the treatment of severe posttraumatic osteoarthritis of the tibiotalar joint. Patients considered for an ankle arthrodesis were offered joint distraction with Ilizarov external fixation. A total of 11 patients had Ilizarov joint distraction for at least 3 months, along with measurement of intra-articular hydrostatic pressure. Patients were allowed full weight bearing on the affected extremity starting a "few days" after application. Retrospective review showed that distraction for 3 months resulted in clinical improvement in pain and mobility for a mean of 2 years, with an increase in joint space. Measurement of the intra-articular hydrostatic pressure during distraction and weight bearing produced values almost identical to those showing improved osteoarthritic cartilage in vitro. These researchers suggested that the intermittent hydrostatic pressure induced by the distraction with weight bearing, in combination with the absence of mechanical stress, may stimulate actual repair of osteoarthritic cartilage.[7] This small retrospective study stimulated further research and an increased interest in joint distraction for ankle arthritis. van Valburg, van Roermund, and their colleagues[5,6,8,21–23] have since been at the forefront in the work of ankle joint distraction for the treatment of ankle arthritis.

SCIENTIFIC BASIS

The surgical technique of arthrodiastasis for arthritis is predicated on the belief that the osteoarthritic joint has some reparative capability when the mechanical stress of the joint is decreased for an appropriate duration of time. The unique articular characteristics of the ankle joint seem especially suited for this technique. The ankle joint cartilage is exposed to higher loads per unit surface area than the hip and knee with walking. Accordingly, the ankle joint cartilage has different thickness and tensile properties than the knee and hip.[24] This difference in biochemical and biomechanical properties may afford the ankle joint a greater capacity for repair, as reported in a recent study comparing cadaveric knee and ankle joints. When compared with the knee, the ankle joint extracellular matrix was found to have a significantly higher proteoglycan content, lower water content, and lower hydraulic permeability. These properties result in higher compressive stiffness of the ankle cartilage. Chondrocytes of the ankle joint were also found to have a decreased response to known catabolic factors. Furthermore, ankle chondrocytes were shown to have an increased response to anabolic agents and, in response to damage, synthesized proteoglycans and collagen at a higher rate than that found in knee chondrocytes.[11]

Arthrodiastasis is believed to optimize the nutrition and reparative properties of the articular cartilage by mechanical unloading of the joint and restoration of intermittent intra-articular hydrostatic fluid pressure changes. Applying hinges to the external fixator construct allows joint motion under distraction and has been shown to have a positive effect on the joint fluid pressure.[20] Similarly, when using a circular ring external fixator for joint distraction, intra-articular hydrostatic fluid pressure levels are restored with repetitive weight bearing as a result of the flexibility of the frame and the stiffness of the joint capsule.[7] In vitro studies have demonstrated that intermittent hydrostatic pressure changes applied to human osteoarthritic cartilage significantly enhanced the synthesis of matrix proteoglycan.[9] In addition, stretching of the periarticular nerve fiber endings was found to occur with joint distraction, potentially supporting a mechanism for pain relief.[8]

An in vivo canine study further experimentally supports this theory.[23] Osteoarthritic canine knees were created by transection of the anterior cruciate ligament. The dogs were then divided into three groups: the first group had no treatment; the second group underwent Ilizarov articulating joint distraction with hinges; and the third group received nonarticulating Ilizarov joint distraction, blocking motion at the joint. During exercise, the intra-articular fluid pressure of the treatment groups was measured. No change was found in the nonarticulating group; however, the articulating distraction group had fluid pressure levels measuring from 3 to 12 kPa with joint movement, comparable to the known levels that have been shown to be beneficial in vitro on human osteoarthritic cartilage. Furthermore, a reduction in synovial inflammation and changes in proteoglycan metabolism that resembled the contralateral normal knee were found in the articulated group. In contrast, after nonarticulating distraction, proteoglycan metabolism was found to be significantly different when compared with the contralateral knee. Fourteen weeks after the application of distraction, the articular cartilage was histologically examined. Although cartilage repair was not found in this study, the results do support the positive metabolic changes caused by articulated joint distraction. These researchers also believed that given a longer follow-up, histologic changes showing cartilage repair would have been present.[23]

The unloading of the periarticular subchondral bone by means of joint distraction is another proposed mechanism leading to cartilage growth and repair. A recent study indicates that subchondral bone plays a crucial role in the development and progression of osteoarthritis.[17] The decrease in subchondral bone density, as suggested by radiographs taken after joint distraction, may allow for decreased stiffness and greater stress absorption, potentially resulting in lower stress on the overlying cartilage. Growth factors in the subchondral bone known to be involved in cartilage growth and repair may also be released with the bone turnover facilitated by offloading.[10] Finally, by halting the progressive changes of the subchondral bone caused by abnormal loading, the potential deleterious effects on the articular cartilage are halted. The cartilage repair process may protect the subchondral bone from loading, however, and thus contribute to decreasing the subchondral bone density.

CLINICAL STUDIES

In 1995, the first retrospective review on distraction arthroplasty of the ankle joint for posttraumatic arthritis was published (**Table 1**).[7] Eleven patients with a mean age of 35 years who were candidates for ankle arthrodesis underwent joint distraction of 5 mm maintained by an Ilizarov external fixator for a mean of 3 months. Full weight bearing a few days after surgery was allowed, and hinges were applied to the fixator between 6 and 12 weeks after surgery to allow for flexion and extension of the ankle joint. At a mean follow-up of 20 months, all patients had decreased pain, with 5 being completely pain-free. Range of motion improved in 6 of the 11 patients, and of the 6 patients with radiographs available at follow-up, 3 (50%) showed an increase in joint space.[7]

After this study, results of ankle joint distraction for severe osteoarthritis were reported in a prospective series with a 2-year follow-up of 17 patients (10 male and 7 female).[22] All subjects (mean age of 39.6 years) were graded prospectively and at yearly intervals after treatment by means of a standardized clinical examination, including physical examination, a functional ability questionnaire, a pain scale, joint mobility, and radiographic evaluation. Standard application of an Ilizarov circular external fixator was performed, enabling tibiotalar joint distraction. Thirteen patients underwent operative arthroscopy before fixator application with removal of intra-articular fibrosis and osteophytes if necessary. Distraction of the joint was performed with a frequency of two times (0.5 mm) daily until a total distraction of 5 mm was reached. In 7 patients, equinus position was corrected in combination with distraction. One week after surgery, full weight bearing was allowed. Joint distraction was performed for 3 months. Four of the 17 patients failed to show significant improvement with joint distraction, and ankle fusion was performed within the first year. Of the remaining 13 patients, significant improvement in more than two thirds was demonstrated by physical examination, a functional ability questionnaire, and a pain scale. These results were shown to be progressive, with further improvement noted at year 2 of follow-up. On average, joint mobility and radiographic joint space were maintained. The investigators concluded that these findings substantiate Ilizarov joint distraction as a promising treatment for severe ankle arthritis.[22]

In 2002, the work continued when Marijnissen and colleagues[5] reported the results of their multicenter prospective study. Fifty-seven patients (mean age of 44 years) with severe refractory arthritic ankle pain who had previously been considered for arthrodesis were enrolled and followed for a mean of 2.8 years. Operative arthroscopic debridement to enable plantigrade foot positioning necessary for distraction was performed in 35 of the 57 patients before application of the Ilizarov external fixator. Standard techniques for application, distraction, and weight bearing were used as described previously. At 1 year, 11 of the 57 patients were lost to follow-up and 8 withdrew from the study because of persistent pain that required arthrodesis. Of the remaining 38 patients, a statistically significant clinical condition improvement by 120% ($P<.0001$) was found, with a significant decrease in pain score by 38% ($P<.0001$), a significant increase in function score by 69% ($P<.0001$), and an increase in joint mobility by 8% (not significant). The improvement in these parameters increased over time, with a progressive clinical benefit maintained during the entire period of follow-up. The patient sample size, however, progressively decreased from 38 at year 1 to 27, 19, 10, 7, 6, and 1 for years 2 through 7, respectively. A total of 13 patients required arthrodesis, including 5 patients from years 2 through 7, with the remaining patients lost to follow-up.

Additionally, radiographs from 17 of the 24 patients from one center were available for evaluation. In 12 of these patients, ankle joint space was decreased before surgery greater than 10% when compared with the contralateral ankle. At 1 year of follow-up after distraction, the average joint space was increased by 17% in these patients, and progressive improvement was seen at 3 years with an additional joint space increase of 10% compared with year 1. Of the remaining 5 patients with pretreatment joint space narrowing less than 10% when compared with the contralateral ankle, no significant change in joint space occurred over time. In those patients with subchondral sclerosis evident before surgery, an average decrease in sclerosis of 10% was measured radiographically at 1 year and a tendency toward improvement over time was demonstrated.

This same article also reported the results of a randomized controlled trial of 17 patients who had severe ankle osteoarthritis.[5] Nine patients (mean age of 44 years) were randomized to undergo Ilizarov joint distraction, and 8 patients (mean age of 45 years) were randomized to undergo arthroscopic joint debridement. Arthroscopic ankle evaluation was performed on all patients before surgery, with debridement of 7 of the 9 patients in the fixator group and all 8 patients in the debridement group. At 1 year of follow-up, the distraction group had similar results to the open prospective Ilizarov joint distraction study reported in the same article, with significant improvements in pain score, function, and clinical status. Three of 8 patients in the debridement group did not reach 1 year of follow-up because of severe pain. These patients were considered to have treatment failure and subsequently underwent joint distraction. Significantly less profound results were found in the debridement group with regard to pain, clinical status, and mobility as compared with the distraction group. The combined results from these studies "prove the concept of joint distraction as a treatment for osteoarthritis" according to Marijnissen and colleagues.[5]

The prolonged benefit of Ilizarov joint distraction in the treatment of ankle arthritis was addressed in 2005 by Ploegmakers and colleagues.[6] Twenty-two patients

Table 1
Clinical studies review

Study	Study Type	Sample Size and Gender	Age (Years)	Follow-Up	Outcome
van Valburg et al (1995)	Retrospective Ilizarov fixator Distraction of ankle joint 5 mm for 15 ± 3 months	n = 11 (4 F and 7 M)	35 ± 13	20 ± 6 months WB after application Hinges applied between 6 and 12 weeks Flexion of ankle allowed	Pain decrease in all 5 of 11 patients pain-free ROM improved in 6 of 11 patients 6 patients had radiographs available 3 of 6 patients had joint spice widening
van Valburg et al (1999)	Prospective Ilizarov fixator Distraction 5 mm for 3 months Arthroscopic debridement before distraction (13 of 17 patients)	n = 17 (7 F and 10 M)	39.6 ± 11.4	1 and 2 years 4 patients had no improvement before first year f/u and required arthrodesis	13 of 17 patients had significant improvement in physical examination, function, and pain Progressive improvement in year 2
Marijnissen et al (2002)	Prospective Ilizarov fixator Distraction 5 mm for 3 months Arthroscopic debridement before distraction (35 of 37 patients)	n = 57 (6 F and 31 M)	44 ± 11	2.8 ± 0.3 years At year 1 f/u, n = 38 8 patients withdrew from the study because of pain in f/u years 2–7 n = 27, 19, 10, 7, 6, and 1	n = 38 at 1 year Significant improvement in pain, function, and clinical condition increased over time 13 patients required arthrodesis over 7 years of f/u
	Prospective randomized All patients examined arthroscopically (first group) Ilizarov distraction 5 mm for 3 months Arthroscopic debridement in 7 of 9 patients (second group) Arthroscopic debridement control	Exp. n = 9 (3 F and 6 M) Control n = 8 (3 F and 5 M)	44 ± 10 45 ± 10	1 year	f/u for 9 of 9 patients at 1 year Results similar to open prospective study, progressive improvement with time Debridement group: 3 of 8 failed at 1 year Significantly less profound clinical results

Study	Procedure	n	Age	Follow-up / Methods	Results
Inda et al (2003)	Retrospective hinged Ilizarov distraction 9 mm for 3 months Debridement/osteotomy/soft tissue release as necessary	n = 9	Not given	1 year WB immediately Hinges locked for 2 weeks and then ROM	All patients had improvement radiographically, wider joint space, satisfaction, and improvement in pain
Ploegmakers et al (2005)	Retrospective Ilizarov joint distraction 5 mm for 15 ± 3 weeks	n = 22 (8 F and 14 M)	37 ± 11	7 years 3 different questionnaires used to evaluate pain, function, clinical status, and mobility	6 (27%) of 22 patients failed treatment 5 patients underwent arthrodesis and 1 had Sudek's atrophy 16 (73%) of 22 patients had significant improvement in all clinical parameters evaluated
Paley and Lamb (2005)	Retrospective hinged Ilizarov distraction for 4 months Osteotomy/debridement/soft tissue release to restore anatomy and ROM	n = 20	Not given	2–16 years	18 of 20 patients had good or excellent results No patients required ankle arthrodesis

Abbreviations: Exp, experimental; F, female; f/u, follow-up; M, male; ROM, range of motion.

(mean age of 37 years) who had been treated with Ilizarov joint distraction were retrospectively followed for 7 years. At the time of evaluation, 6 of these 22 patients were judged to have treatment failure. Five patients underwent arthrodesis because of persisting pain, and 1 patient developed Sudeck's atrophy. The remaining 16 (73%) patients showed significant improvement in all clinical parameters observed based on three standardized evaluation approaches.[6]

Inda and colleagues[25] reported on nine articulated joint distractions of the ankle using a hinged Ilizarov external fixator. Additional procedures, including supramalleolar osteotomy, ankle arthroscopy, and anterior ankle arthrotomy with debridement, were performed at the same setting when needed to restore normal joint anatomy. The articulated fixator was applied, and the ankle was initially distracted approximately 2 mm. Gradual distraction of 1 mm/d in four separate daily adjustments was prescribed to achieve a total distraction of 9 mm. Patients were allowed to bear weight immediately, and the hinges were locked for 2 weeks, after which ankle range of joint motion was initiated. At an average follow-up of 1 year, all patients had radiographic improvement in joint space and reported satisfaction, improvement in pain, and increased ankle dorsiflexion; however, the overall range of motion did not improve. Similarly, in 2005, Paley and Lamm[26] reported the preliminary results of the first 20 ankle joints treated according to their technique. After all blocking osteophytes were removed, all joint contractures were released, and correction of osseous alignment of the ankle joint was restored, a hinged circular ring external fixator was applied. The fixator was kept in place for 4 months, weight bearing was allowed as tolerated, and range of motion at the ankle was encouraged. With a follow-up ranging from 2 to 16 years, 18 of the 20 patients had a good or excellent result, with no patients requiring arthrodesis.

The most common complications encountered in ankle joint distraction include superficial pin site infection and irritation.[27] Treatment consists of local wound care and oral antibiotics. Occasionally, hardware failure occurs, necessitating removal or replacement of pins or wires. Neurovascular injury can occur with improper pin or wire placement or with overdistraction of the frame. Failure to relieve pain is another potential complication that has been encountered, with treatment consisting of frame removal and eventual ankle arthrodesis. Other complications common to all reconstructive foot and ankle surgery exist.

RECOMMENDED INDICATION AND TECHNIQUE

Ideal candidates who might benefit from ankle joint distraction therapy are those patients who have posttraumatic arthritis and are younger than 45 years of age. The major indication for treatment is pain severe enough to consider ankle arthrodesis. Arthroscopic evaluation and debridement of the ankle joint osteophytes have been performed in most clinical studies and are recommended before external fixator application. Open restoration of the articular surface with osteotomies or release of soft tissue contractures should be performed when needed to allow for neutral alignment of the foot and ankle. Circular ring external fixation should be used for distraction of the ankle while allowing the patient to be weight bearing. Sequential distraction of the joint after application to a total of 5 mm should be maintained during treatment. Range of motion of the ankle joint during distraction has also been shown to be beneficial and supports the use of hinges in the fixator. All current studies recommend treatment for at least 3 months, with adjustments as necessary to maintain distraction at 5 mm.

Frame application begins with placement of the proximal ring and half pins and is performed without a tourniquet. A twist plate with a one-hole post is attached anteriorly to the proximal ring before application. The one-hole post marks the anterior midline of the proximal ring and is used as a reference. The distal half pin is ideally placed 6 cm proximal to the medial malleolus, on the anterior tibial crest, and just medial to the tibialis anterior tendon. This pin is predrilled while checking intraoperative lateral radiographs to ensure perpendicular placement to the tibial shaft. The half pin is inserted with bicortical purchase and attached to the proximal ring in the most distal hole of a three-hole post, usually two holes medial to the anterior twist plate. Orthogonal placement of the ring to the axis of the tibia is ensured before tightening all connections (**Fig. 2**). The proximal half pin is then positioned on the anterior-medial border of the tibia to obtain multiplanar fixation. Using a three-hole post as a guide, placing the post approximately three ring holes medially from the first post, the half pin is predrilled and bicortically inserted (**Fig. 3**). After ensuring orthogonal ring placement with radiographs, all connections are tightened.

To ensure proper positioning of hinges, a reference wire is placed to visualize the ankle joint axis. Using fluoroscopic assistance, a smooth k-wire is inserted through the talus from the tip of the lateral malleolus aiming for the tip of the medial malleolus (**Fig. 4**). A lateral radiograph is taken to ensure placement of the guidewire in the center of the talar body. Medial and lateral articulated threaded rods are then attached to the frame. Using the reference wire as a guide, the threaded rods are positioned to allow the center point of the hinge to intersect perfectly with the wire. Typically, a 150-mm threaded rod and hinge assembly is needed medially and 120 mm laterally. The rods are then tightened to the proximal ring, paying careful attention to make sure that the square nut is distal to the ring and enough threaded rod is proximal to the ring to allow for desired distraction (**Fig. 5**). The reference wire is then removed.

A closed foot-plate is constructed by securing a four-hole L-plate to the most distal hole of each arm in the foot-plate. These L-plates are then connected through their most proximal hole by a threaded rod containing a three-hole female post as shown. The foot-plate is attached to the articulated rods, with the foot and ankle held in neutral

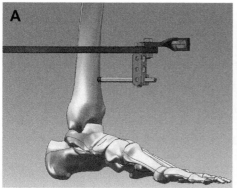
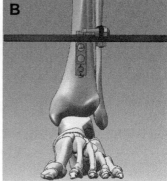

Fig. 2. Orthogonal alignment of the proximal ring connected to the distal half-pin (*A*). A one-hole post connected to the anterior twist plate on the proximal ring is placed anteriorly midline and used as a reference for alignment (*B*). (*Courtesy of* Small Bone Innovations, Inc., New York, NY; with permission.)

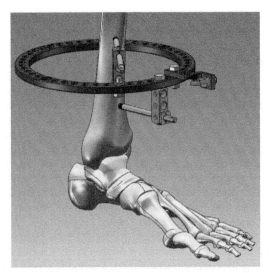

Fig. 3. Distal and proximal half-pins are oriented to ensure multiplanar fixation of proximal ring. (*Courtesy of* Small Bone Innovations, Inc., New York, NY; with permission.)

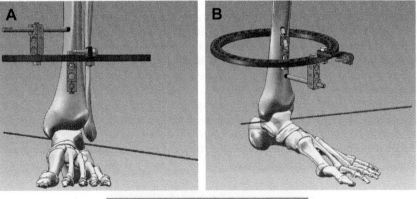

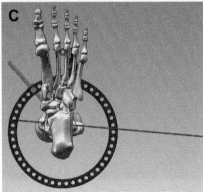

Fig. 4. (*A–C*) Placement of the ankle joint axis reference wire from the tip of the lateral malleolus to the tip of the medial malleolus. (*Courtesy of* Small Bone Innovations, Inc., New York, NY; with permission.)

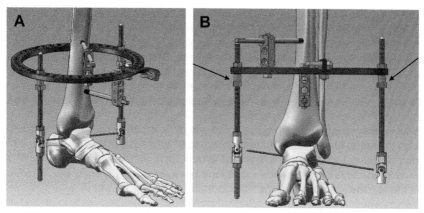

Fig. 5. Attachment of articulated threaded rods to the proximal ring. (*A*) Midpoint of each hinge is aligned with the axis guide. (*B*) Arrows demonstrate square nut placement distal to the proximal ring to facilitate future distraction. (*Courtesy of* Small Bone Innovations, Inc., New York, NY; with permission.)

alignment. The foot-plate should fit with at least two finger breaths of clearance around all sides, and the plantar surface of the foot should extend approximately 1 inch beyond the plate to facilitate weight bearing. After the rods are connected, the motion of the foot-plate should be smooth; if not, the rods and hinges need adjustment (**Fig. 6**).

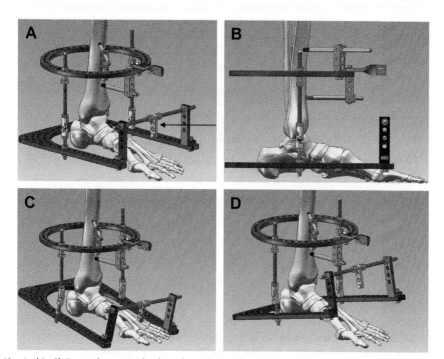

Fig. 6. (*A, B*) Foot-plate attached to threaded rods with the foot in neutral alignment. The arrow demonstrates three-hole female post placement in the middle of a threaded rod connecting two four-hole L-plates. (*C, D*) Range-of-motion evaluation to ensure proper placement of hinges. (*Courtesy of* Small Bone Innovations, Inc., New York, NY; with permission.)

The foot-plate is then secured to the foot, first by inserting an olive wire transversely through the posterior calcaneus laterally to medially within the calcaneal safe zone. The wire is tensioned and attached to the foot-plate. Another olive wire is placed medially to laterally through the talar neck. The wire is placed with fluoroscopic guidance and must exist anterior to the fibula. The frame is built up to secure the wire with posts, and the wire is tensioned. Finally, a third smooth wire is placed in the calcaneus posteriorly to medially from an anteriorl-to-lateral direction, is tensioned, and is secured to the frame (**Fig. 7**).

A threaded rod is then slid through the one-hole post in the proximal ring twist plate toward the knee. At the distal end of the threaded rod, a square nut and regular nut are placed. The distal end of the rod is threaded through the three-hole female post on the foot-plate and tightened with the nut. Range of motion of the ankle is evaluated with the anterior threaded rod in place. The foot and ankle are placed in neutral position, and square nuts are tightened on adjacent sides of the one-hole post to lock the frame in this position (**Fig. 8**).

With the frame locked in neutral position, the hex nuts on the proximal side of the tibial ring attached to the threaded hinge and rod construct are loosened. The proximal square nut on the anterior threaded rod is also loosened. The frame is then distracted by rotating the square nuts on the distal side of the tibial ring of each rod. Tightening or clockwise rotation of each square nut one full rotation equals 1 mm of distraction. Alternating distraction of medial, lateral, and anterior rods 1 mm at a time is repeated until a total of 2 mm of ankle joint distraction is obtained (**Fig. 9**). This is evaluated clinically and radiographically. When satisfied with distraction, all frame connections are tightened. The patient is admitted for observation and

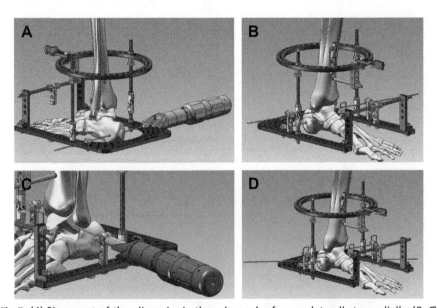

Fig. 7. (*A*) Placement of the olive wire in the calcaneal safe zone laterally to medially. (*B, C*) Olive wire placed in the neck/body of the talus just anterior to the fibula medially to laterally and attached to the foot-plate with posts. This ensures that distraction only occurs at the ankle joint. (*D*) Smooth wire inserted in the calcaneus posteriorly to medially to an anterior-to-lateral direction and secured to the foot-plate. (*Courtesy of* Small Bone Innovations, Inc., New York, NY; with permission.)

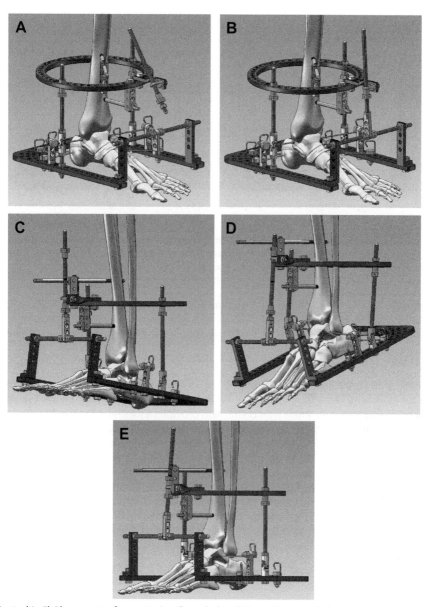

Fig. 8. (*A, B*) Placement of an anterior threaded rod through a one-hole post in the anterior twist plate and into the female end of the three-hole post distally. (*C, D*) Range of motion is evaluated with the anterior threaded rod in place. (*E*) Frame is locked in neutral alignment with square nuts securing the anterior threaded rod on adjacent sides of the one-hole post. (*Courtesy of* Small Bone Innovations, Inc., New York, NY; with permission.)

allowed full weight bearing of the affected extremity on the first postoperative day. Gradual distraction of 1 mm/d in four separate daily adjustments is prescribed to achieve a total distraction of 5 mm. At 2 weeks, the patient is instructed on adjustment of the anterior threaded rod and range of motion of the ankle is begun

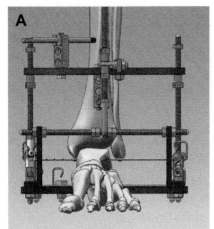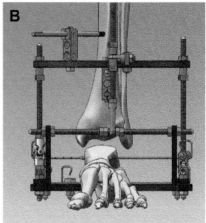

Fig. 9. (*A*) Loosening of the proximal nuts on the articulated and anterior threaded rods. (*B*) Distraction of the ankle joint; one full turn of each square nut equals 1 mm of distraction. (*Courtesy of* Small Bone Innovations, Inc., New York, NY; with permission.)

gradually. The frame is applied for 3 months, with adjustments made as necessary to maintain distraction and stability.

SUMMARY

Arthritis of the ankle joint is a progressive and disabling disorder that primarily occurs in young patients secondary to trauma. When nonoperative treatment fails in patients who have ankle arthritis, ankle joint distraction provides a joint-sparing treatment alternative, avoiding the potential complications associated with ankle arthrodesis or joint replacement. Scientific data demonstrate a healing potential present in osteoarthritic ankle cartilage. Furthermore, research supports positive biochemical and biomechanical intra-articular changes associated with joint distraction, facilitating an environment for cartilage repair. Multiple clinical studies have demonstrated improvement in symptoms and positive radiologic changes, validating joint distraction in the treatment of ankle arthritis. Continued research is needed to evaluate this technique further; however, current data support joint distraction as a viable treatment for ankle arthritis in the younger patient with a congruent joint.

REFERENCES

1. Glazebrook M, Daniels T, Younger A, et al. Comparison of health-related quality of life between patients with end-stage ankle and hip arthrosis. J Bone Joint Surg Am 2008;90(3):499–505.
2. Saltzman CL, Salamon ML, Blanchard GM, et al. Epidemiology of ankle arthritis: report of a consecutive series of 639 patients from a tertiary orthopaedic center. Iowa Orthop J 2005;25:44–6.
3. Buchner M, Sabo D. Ankle fusion attributable to posttraumatic arthrosis: a long-term followup of 48 patients. Clin Orthop Relat Res 2003;406:155–64.
4. Fuchs S, Sandmann C, Skwara A, et al. Quality of life 20 years after arthrodesis of the ankle: a study of adjacent joints. J Bone Joint Surg Br 2003;85(7):994–8.

5. Marijnissen AC, van Roermund PM, van Melkebeek J, et al. Clinical benefit of joint distraction in the treatment of severe osteoarthritis of the ankle: proof of concept in an open prospective study and in a randomized controlled study. Arthritis Rheum 2002;46(11):2893–902.
6. Ploegmakers JJ, van Roermund PM, van Melkebeek J, et al. Prolonged clinical benefit from joint distraction in the treatment of ankle osteoarthritis. Osteoarthr Cartil 2005;13(7):582–8.
7. van Valburg AA, van Roermund PM, Lammens J, et al. Can Ilizarov joint distraction delay the need for an arthrodesis of the ankle? A preliminary report. J Bone Joint Surg Br 1995;77(5):720–5.
8. van Valburg AA, van Roy HL, Lafeber FP, et al. Beneficial effects of intermittent fluid pressure of low physiological magnitude on cartilage and inflammation in osteoarthritis. An in vitro study. J Rheumatol 1998;25(3):515–20.
9. Lafeber FP, Veldhuijzen JP, Vanroy JL, et al. Intermittent hydrostatic compressive force stimulates exclusively the proteoglycan synthesis of osteoarthritic human cartilage. Br J Rheumatol 1992;31(7):437–42.
10. Lafeber FP, Intema F, Van Roermund PM, et al. Unloading joints to treat osteoarthritis, including joint distraction. Curr Opin Rheumatol 2006;18(5):519–25.
11. Kuettner KE, Cole AA. Cartilage degeneration in different human joints. Osteoarthr Cartil 2005;13(2):93–103.
12. Carter DR, Beaupre GS, Wong M, et al. The mechanobiology of articular cartilage development and degeneration. Clin Orthop Relat Res 2004;(427 Suppl):S69–77.
13. Goldring MB, Goldring SR. Osteoarthritis. J Cell Physiol 2007;213(3):626–34.
14. Roos EM. Joint injury causes knee osteoarthritis in young adults. Curr Opin Rheumatol 2005;17(2):195–200.
15. Furman BD, Olson SA, Guilak F. The development of posttraumatic arthritis after articular fracture. J Orthop Trauma 2006;20(10):719–25.
16. Martin JA, Brown TD, Heiner AD, et al. Chondrocyte senescence, joint loading and osteoarthritis. Clin Orthop Relat Res 2004;(427 Suppl):S96–103.
17. Lajeunesse D, Reboul P. Subchondral bone in osteoarthritis: a biologic link with articular cartilage leading to abnormal remodeling. Curr Opin Rheumatol 2003; 15(5):628–33.
18. Volkov MV, Oganesian OV. Restoration of function in the knee and elbow with a hinge-distractor apparatus. J Bone Joint Surg Am 1975;57(5):591–600.
19. Judet R, Judet T. [The use of a hinge distraction apparatus after arthrolysis and arthroplasty (author's translation)]. Rev Chir Orthop Reparatrice Appar Mot 1978; 64(5):353–65 [in French].
20. Aldegheri R, Trivella G, Saleh M. Articulated distraction of the hip. Conservative surgery for arthritis in young patients. Clin Orthop Relat Res 1994;(301):94–101.
21. van Roermund PM, van Valburg AA, Duivemann E, et al. Function of stiff joints may be restored by Ilizarov joint distraction. Clin Orthop Relat Res 1998;(348): 220–7.
22. van Valburg AA, van Roermund PM, Marijnissen AC, et al. Joint distraction in treatment of osteoarthritis: a two-year follow-up of the ankle. Osteoarthr Cartil 1999;7(5):474–9.
23. van Valburg AA, van Roermund PM, Marijnissen AC. Joint distraction in treatment of osteoarthritis (II): effects on cartilage in a canine model. Osteoarthr Cartil 2000; 8(1):1–8.
24. El-Khoury GY, Alliman KJ, Lundberg HJ, et al. Cartilage thickness in cadaveric ankles: measurement with double-contrast multi-detector row CT arthrography versus MR imaging. Radiology 2004;233(3):768–73.

25. Inda DJ, Blyakher A, O'Malley MJ, et al. Distraction arthroplasty for the ankle using the Ilizarov frame. Tech Foot Ankle Surg 2003;2(4):249–53.
26. Paley D, Lamm BM. Ankle joint distraction. Foot Ankle Clin 2005;10(4):685–98.
27. van Roermund PM, Lafeber FP, Marijnissen AC. Joint distraction in the treatment of ankle arthritis. In: Rozbruch SR, Ilizarov S, editors. Functional reconstruction. New York: Informa Healthcare USA; 2007. p. 273–8.

Supramalleolar Osteotomy

Shannon M. Rush, DPM, FACFAS

KEYWORDS

• Ankle deformity • Malunion • Osteotomy • Correction

Realignment osteotomy of the distal tibia is a valuable surgical procedure for the treatment of distal tibial malalignment resulting from posttraumatic malunion, physeal disturbances, congenital and metabolic diseases, and degenerative arthritis.[1–11] The purpose of supramalleolar osteotomy (SMO) is to preserve the ankle and foot from articular degeneration and biomechanical dysfunction by restoring the joint orientation and axial alignment of the ankle and hind foot. Juxta-articular malalignment of the distal tibia often results in hind foot and forefoot compensation, which, over time, creates predictable patterns of joint degeneration and pain. Gait disturbances can have detrimental effects on the ipsilateral hip, knee, and spine. Small degrees of malalignment are well tolerated, given that there is no concomitant stiffness or arthritis in the adjacent hind foot joints.[12,13] Heywood[10] described SMO in patients who had rheumatoid arthritis and secondary deformity to restore a plantargrade foot and preserve hind foot motion. Takakura and collegues[8,9] described SMO for the treatment of posttraumatic arthritis and malunion. These researchers were able to demonstrate the restorative influence that SMO has on the articular cartilage. In a small series of hemophilic ankle valgus deformity resulting from recurring hemarthrosis, Pearce and colleagues[11] demonstrated that realignment osteotomy preserved function and eliminated the need for need for secondary reconstructive surgery at 9 years of follow-up.

In addition, limb length inequality, restriction of normal joint motion, soft tissue contracture, and compensatory adaptation in the foot are all potential surgical considerations that require evaluation when planning an osteotomy near the ankle joint. Severe scarring, previous soft tissue transfer, or skin grafting may alter the surgical approach and influence the type or location of osteotomy. The clinical and radiographic evaluation of deformity and execution of corrective osteotomy have been described in a comprehensive way by Paley[14,15] and Paley and Lamm.[14–16] Using concepts of vector trigonometry, corrective SMO can be evaluated and treated with predictable results. A thorough clinical evaluation, including physical examination,

Camino Division, Department of Orthopedics, Palo Alto Medical Foundation, 701 East El Camino Real, Mountain View, CA 94040, USA
E-mail address: rushdoc@gmail.com

Clin Podiatr Med Surg 26 (2009) 245–257
doi:10.1016/j.cpm.2008.12.008
0891-8422/08/$ – see front matter © 2009 Elsevier Inc. All rights reserved.

stance and gait evaluation, radiographic planning, and, in some instances, manual stress views of the ankle and subtalar joint, is necessary.[16]

INDICATIONS

The most frequently encountered indication for SMO in the author's practice is for posttraumatic malunion and secondary degenerative arthritis. Often, only a portion of the articular surface of the joint is involved, and corrective osteotomy can salvage the remaining articular surface by redistribution of pathologic wear patterns on the joint. Takakura and colleagues[8] demonstrated that focal degenerative wear patterns could be positively affected with regeneration of fibrocartilage by arthroscopic debridement and SMO. The importance of restoring axis alignment and joint orientation is critical for eliminating abnormal degenerative wear patterns on the articular surface and diminishing secondary subtalar and forefoot compensation.[17,18] Chronic lateral ankle instability resulting from ankle varus is difficult to correct with calcaneal osteotomy and lateral ankle ligament reconstruction. Varus chondral wear patterns often lead to a recurrence of varus instability. Calcaneal osteotomy often fails to realign the mechanical axis of the limb adequately, leading to failure of the reconstruction. Valgus corrective osteotomy can more appropriately address the varus joint orientation of the tibiotalar joint (**Fig. 1**). Valgus SMO is also indicated in the cavovarus foot. Hind foot osteotomy and midfoot correction are often inadequate to correct the intrinsic varus ankle joint orientation. These adaptive wear patterns develop over many years and may not be as obvious as the foot deformity, although they are just as important to adequate deformity correction. Valgus corrective osteotomy can be a helpful adjunctive procedure to achieve rectus alignment (**Fig. 2**).

Malpositioned ankle arthrodeses can lead to significant degenerative changes in the subtalar and midtarsal joints with alteration in the ground reactive forces (GRFs) generated in the limb. Sagittal plane malalignment can lead to degeneration of the midtarsal joint and generate recurvatum thrust on the knee. Corrective osteotomy for ankle arthrodesis malunion is directed at restoring a plantargrade foot and realigning the tibiocalcaneal axis (**Fig. 3**). Growth plate disturbances from fracture or infection can result in significant secondary deformity. Often, limb length inequality is an additional consideration in these cases, and planning must take excessive shortening into account. McNicol and colleagues[5] and Scheffer and Peterson[6] demonstrated the use of SMO for congenital deformity in children. McNicol and colleagues[5] used a derotational osteotomy in children with complex equinovarus deformity and external tibial torsion. Scheffer and Peterson[6] described an opening wedge osteotomy to correct deformity and restore length. Best and Daniels[18] treated a small series of four patients who had five opening wedge osteotomies with a Puddu plate (Arthex Inc., Naples, Florida). Autogenous bone was used in all cases, and all osteotomies had healed by 3 months.

BIOMECHANICAL RATIONALE FOR SUPRAMALLEOLAR OSTEOTOMY

Articular cartilage can be adversely affected by malalignment, and chondral wear patterns can develop rapidly with deformity.[17,19] The degree to which the deformity influences clinical symptoms and function depends on several factors, including the degree of motion in the subtalar and midtarsal joint, size of the individual, severity of the index injury, intra-articular fracture patterns, articular incongruity, and age. The available amount of motion in the subtalar joint is not precisely understood and can vary considerably among patients.[20,21] Paley[14] believes that 30° of ankle valgus and 15° of ankle varus can be compensated for with a normal functioning subtalar joint

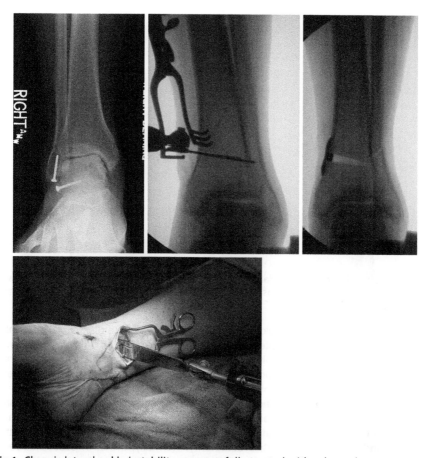

Fig. 1. Chronic lateral ankle instability unsuccessfully treated with calcaneal osteotomy and lateral ligament reconstruction. Unrecognized ankle varus was the underlying cause of recurrent instability. The patient was treated with a metaphyseal opening wedge osteotomy and Puddu plate. The wedge back was filled with ipsilateral calcaneal autograft.

(Fig. 4). Distal tibial valgus deformity is better compensated for than distal tibial varus deformity, because twice as much inversion exists in the subtalar joint than eversion. When the distal tibial deformity exceeds the available frontal plane compensation in the subtalar joint, several clinical scenarios develop. When the amount of ankle varus deformity exceeds the available subtalar eversion, a residual hind foot varus deformity results. This condition creates additional forefoot pronation to maintain a plantargrade foot. The opposite occurs when a distal tibial valgus deformity is incompletely compensated for. Complicating this condition is the progressive development of degenerative stiffness in the subtalar joint, with the inability to compensate for distal tibial deformity. Further, joint axis malalignment causes degenerative articular wear patterns. Tarr and colleagues[19] showed that distal tibial deformity significantly altered the contact location, shape, and magnitude of the tibiotalar contact pressures. Sagittal plane malalignment created the most significant alterations in contact characteristics. Recurvatum (shear deformity) and procurvatum (impingement deformity) of 15° resulted in changes in contact biomechanics of greater than 40%. These cadaver studies showed how deformity near the joint can focus contact pressure to small areas

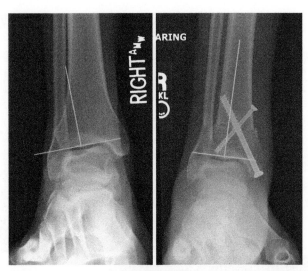

Fig. 2. Cavovarus deformity secondary to Charcot-Marie-Tooth neuropathy. The patient was treated with a lateral calcaneal closing wedge and lateral tibial closing wedge osteotomy.

of the articular surface. This could explain why patients tolerate distal tibial deformity initially and often present only later when painful degenerative articular wear patterns begin in the ankle and subtalar joint. These cadaver studies are difficult to extend into the clinical situation but do correlate with the clinical patterns of articular wear observed. Steffensmeier and colleagues[22,23] demonstrated that the focal areas of the talar dome could be offloaded with shifts in the center of pressure of 1 mm and 1.58 mm with lateral and medial displacement osteotomies of 1 cm, respectively. This shift in the GRF demonstrates the ability to manipulate the GRF acting on the hind foot and ankle with corrective osteotomy. Normally, the GRF passes through the heel and lateral aspect of the ankle joint, creating a valgus torque in the hind foot.[14] The lateral position of the calcaneal axis with respect to the tibial axis explains this mechanical principle. Additionally, abnormal lateral translation (greater than 1 cm) of the calcaneus can cause detrimental hind foot valgus forces. Often, the surgeon encounters a dysfunctional flatfoot with hind foot valgus associated with ankle valgus deformity. This poorly compensated ankle and hind foot valgus predictably leads to posterior tibial tendon dysfunction and deltoid ligament failure over time. Understanding the effects of malalignment of the distal tibia and hind foot is critical to understanding the importance of realignment osteotomy. The foot and ankle surgeon can use these techniques to restore axis alignment and joint orientation and, secondarily, to offload focal degenerative areas of the ankle. The clinical consequence of realignment osteotomy in preserving the tibiotalar joint in the long term is not well documented, although skeletal malalignment must be corrected before arthrodesis or implant arthroplasty.

CLINICAL EVALUATION

A thorough examination of the extremity must include accurate weight-bearing orthogonal radiographs of the ankle and foot, hind foot alignment, and long-leg calcaneal axial views. For conditions that are not attributable to the obvious fracture malunion or physeal injury, full-length standing films are indicated. Close attention

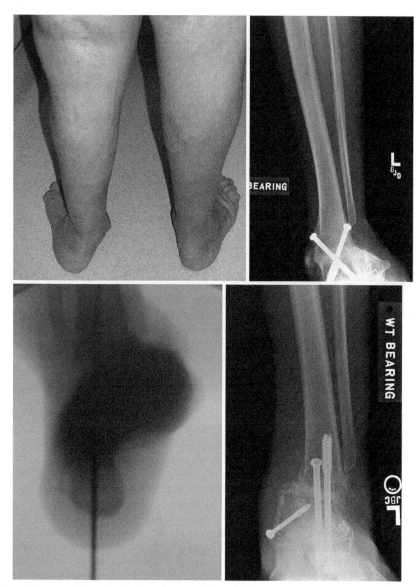

Fig. 3. Valgus ankle arthrodesis malunion. The patient was treated with a medial closing wedge osteotomy through the fusion mass to realign the calcaneal axis to the axis of the tibia. A derotational midfoot osteotomy also was required to maintain a plantargrade forefoot.

must be given to the subtalar joint when planning a correctional osteotomy. Adaptive compensation for a distal tibial deformity may result in stiffness or degenerative arthrosis in the hind foot. Frontal plane corrective osteotomies may realign the ankle joint but unmask adaptive deformity in the subtalar joint, which may be poorly tolerated because of stiffness or arthrosis. Rotational alignment can be assessed on examination with the femoral foot angle. Joint stiffness and arthrosis, which is less objective and often more subtle than radiographic parameters, must be evaluated and included

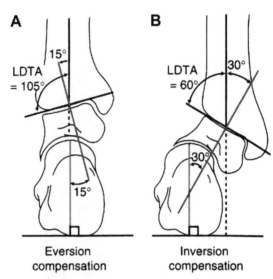

Fig. 4. (*A*) Distal tibial varus of 15° is compensated for with subtalar eversion. (*B*) Distal tibial valgus of 30° is compensated for with subtalar inversion. Note the lateral translation of the calcaneus with respect to the tibial axis in valgus deformity. (*From* Paley D. Principles of deformity correction. Berlin: Springer-Verlag; 2003, p. 574; with permission.)

in the planning process. Diagnostic injections are often useful to confirm painful arthrosis.

Soft tissue adaptation is usually the rule with long-standing deformity. For optimal correction and joint motion after correctional osteotomy, soft tissue releases are usually required. Achilles tendon lengthening or gastrocnemius is the most common adjunctive procedure used, especially with sagittal plane deformity correction. Hind foot tendon rebalancing, such as flexor digitorum longus augmentation of the posterior tibial tendon and peroneus longus–to–peroneus brevis augmentation, can help to stabilize and restore motor function to the hind foot. It is important to record a complete muscle inventory to ensure that previous trauma or periarticular fibrosis has not diminished motor function to any significant degree.

Neural structures, most notably the tibial nerve, are at risk for traction or compression neuropraxic injuries with certain SMOs. Correction of varus, procurvatum, equinus, or internal rotation places the tibial nerve at risk for traction or compression. Prophylactic tarsal tunnel release is generally recommended for any significant degree of correction.[14,16] Care should be taken with release of the tarsal tunnel and porta pedis to decompress the medial and lateral plantar nerves adequately as they pass beneath the abductor hallucis muscle.

Clinical stress examination of the lateral collateral and deltoid complex is a helpful adjunct to determine ligamentous stability. It is common to encounter lateral collateral instability in long-standing varus deformity. Often, secondary soft tissue reconstruction is warranted, which is decided on a case-by-case basis. Manual stress radiographs can guide the surgeon to the appropriate procedure.

Advanced imaging, such as MRI or CT, may also be helpful to evaluate focal articular damage and periarticular pathologic conditions. Arthroscopic debridement of articular injuries and soft tissue impingement should always accompany SMO if clinically warranted. Periarticular spurring is common in long-standing deformity and is as much an adaptation to abnormal joint mechanics as it is degenerative. Lateral plafond spurring in valgus malalignment and medial talar neck spurring in varus malalignment can be addressed with arthroscopic debridement or arthrotomy.

DEFORMITY EVALUATION AND OSTEOTOMY PLANNING

Accurate and reproducible weight-bearing radiographs are important to proper deformity evaluation and deformity planning. Anteroposterior and lateral radiographs of the ankle are the most important films in deformity planning for SMO. The center of the ankle joint and the middiaphyseal line extended to the joint are important parameters to be familiar with. In a rectus angle, the middiaphyseal line should pass through the center of the talus and lateral talar process on the anteroposterior and lateral views, respectively. These landmarks form joint orientation angles, and the lateral orientation angles have been determined. The lateral distal tibial angle (LDTA). (89° ± 3°) and anterior distal tibial angle (ADTA) (80° ± 2°) (**Fig. 5**) are established joint orientation angles.[14] The absolute magnitude of necessary deformity to indicate SMO is not clear and must be taken in the context of clinical condition.

The talocrural angle (82° ± 3.6°)[14] is the angle formed by a line connecting the tip of the medial and lateral malleolus and middiaphyseal line. Deformity in the distal tibia influences this angle, and it is not reliable in such instances. The plafond malleolar (9° ± 4°) angle[14] is the angle formed by the tip of the malleoli and the tibial plafond. This angle is more reliable in the presence of distal tibial deformity (**Fig. 6**).

Long-leg calcaneal axial and hind foot alignment views allow for evaluation of the hind foot and subtalar joint[14] Long-leg calcaneal axial views allow assessment of the subtalar joint and the relation of the calcaneus to the anatomic axis of the tibia. The hind foot alignment view allows evaluation of the calcaneus with respect to the ankle and distal tibia. The calcaneus has a normal lateral translation of 1 cm with respect to the middiaphyseal line.[14] The amount of translation of the calcaneus relative

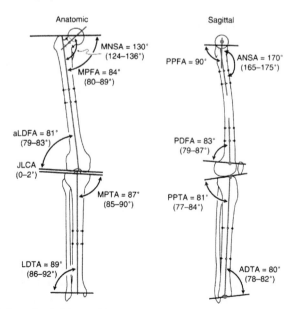

Fig. 5. Normal joint orientation angles and anatomic axes in the frontal and sagittal planes. (*From* Paley D. Principles of deformity correction. Berlin: Springer-Verlag; 2003, p. 9; with permission.)

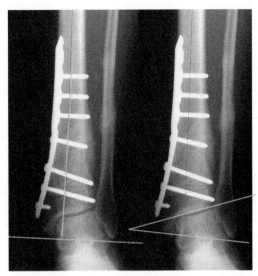

Fig. 6. Determining the relative length of the malleoli can be misleading with distal tibial deformity. The talocrural angle (82° ± 3.6°) is changed with a distal tibial deformity. The plafond malleolar angle (9° ± 4°) is a more accurate way to assess the relative length of the malleoli.

to the tibial axis and the angulation of the calcaneus with respect to the tibia are two important criteria to evaluate. The translational deformity is the most often overlooked residual deformity when performing SMO. Translational or wedge osteotomy can be used to align the calcaneus to the tibial axis properly.

CENTER OF ROTATION OF ANGULATION ANALYSIS

Every deformity has a geometric center that defines the apex of the deformity. This apex is referred to as the center of rotation of angulation (CORA) and serves as an important reference point in osteotomy planning. Generally, the diaphyseal bisection on each side of the deformity defines the location of the CORA. For juxta-articular deformity, a distal middiaphyseal line cannot be drawn accurately. A reference joint orientation angle must be used. The LDTA (89°) and the ADTA (80°) are determined and extended proximally to intersect with the middiaphyseal line proximal to the deformity. The intersection of these lines is the CORA. Often, the level of the CORA is different on anteroposterior and lateral films. This is the result of translation in a different plane from the plane of angulation deformity. Translation is common in fracture malunion deformity of the distal tibia after spiral oblique fractures (**Fig. 7**).

Paley[14] has described a scientific and systematic formula for deformity planning and osteotomy execution. He has described three osteotomy rules that accurately predict the appropriate level of osteotomy and the expected result of the osteotomy based on the location relative to the CORA. Osteotomy rule 1 states that when the osteotomy and axis of correction of angulation (ACA) pass through the CORA, pure angulation correction occurs without translation. Osteotomy rule 2 states that when the ACA is through the CORA but the osteotomy is at a different level, the deformity realigns by angulation and translation at the osteotomy site. Osteotomy rule 3 states that when the osteotomy and ACA are at a level away from the CORA, a translation deformity results. Violation of these principles by improper osteotomy planning may

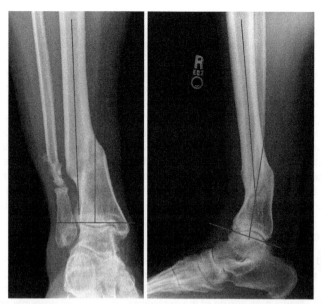

Fig. 7. Recurvatum deformity with medial translation after malunion of a spiral distal tibial fracture. When translation occurs in a plane other than the deformity, the CORA does not correspond on the anteroposterior and lateral films. An osteotomy must correct the recurvatum and medial translation.

introduce iatrogenic deformity, usually in the form of translation. Conversely, knowing that translation can be introduced into the osteotomy, the osteotomy principles can be used in the surgeon's favor when planning deformity correction. For example, a distal tibial malunion with angulation and translation cannot be fully corrected with pure angulation osteotomy. An osteotomy that allows for angulation and translation correction should be used.

The most logical way to approach deformity correction planning is first to understand normal lower limb alignment and joint orientation. It is necessary to define the anatomic axis of the tibia on the anteroposterior and lateral views, to define the middiaphyseal line, and then to extend these distally to the ankle. It is then necessary to draw the LDTA and ADTA, which, when extended proximally, define the CORA. Evaluation of the hind foot alignment with respect to the tibial axis and ankle joint is required. This exercise should define the deformity, level of the CORA, and hind foot position. Clinical examination can determine rotation (femoral foot angle), soft tissue contracture, and ligament instability. This information can then be used to plan the appropriate operation and combination of procedures.

FOCAL DOME OSTEOTOMY

The focal dome osteotomy (FDO) is an osteotomy performed for deformity at or near the ankle joint. The indication for the osteotomy is a deformity that requires angulation correction. The osteotomy describes a portion of the circumference of a circle. Mendicino and collegues[1] described a percutaneous minimally invasive technique that spares periarticular soft tissue dissection and preserves blood supply. The technique is done with the aid of intraoperative imaging. The osteotomy is most appropriate for frontal or sagittal plane correction located at or near the ankle joint. The osteotomy allows for pure angulation correction. No translational correction can be obtained with this technique. In addition, no rotation correction can be achieved.

The surgical technique involves an axis pin at the center of the arc, which is usually placed in the talus or distal tibia near the joint. The center of the pin is ideally placed at the CORA, thereby not introducing any secondary deformity. A Rancho cube placed over the pin allows for circular rotation of the Rancho cube. This rotation describes an arc. The holes in the Rancho cube can be used as a drill guide. Several drill holes placed through the tibia are connected with an osteotome, completing the osteotomy. The fibula also requires an osteotomy, which is performed in an oblique orientation in the same plane and level as the planned osteotomy and allows for fibular translation along the osteotomy. Fixation of the tibial osteotomy can be done in several ways. Given the interdigitation of the osteotomy, percutaneous screws are the most logical method of stabilization (**Fig. 8**). The fibular osteotomy is inherently stable and can be fixed with screws or a lateral plate. Often, the fibula can be left without fixation.

SUPRAMALLEOLAR WEDGE OSTEOTOMY

Opening and closing an osteotomy of the distal tibia is a straightforward technique that affords several advantages. For juxta-articular deformity with the CORA near the joint, the osteotomy can be performed at the CORA. This allows for pure angular correction. The transverse nature of the osteotomy allows small amounts of translation through the osteotomy to restore axis alignment. The transverse design of the osteotomy is inherently stable, and the metaphyseal location of the osteotomy encourages rapid healing. The osteotomy is performed in a limited open fashion with exposure of the base of the osteotomy to be performed. Preoperative templates determine the placement and size of the osteotomy. Osteotomy guide pins can be placed for the desired amount of bone to be removed. The distal pin is placed parallel to the tibial plafond, and the proximal pin is placed perpendicular to the tibial axis. When removed, the area between the converging wires corrects the deformity. Small adjustments in blade orientation result in multiple plane correction. The fibular osteotomy is performed in the same plane as the correction, similar to the FDO. Intraoperative assessment of axial alignment to assess the center of the talus, with respect to the axis of the tibia, in the frontal and sagittal planes is important before definitive fixation. The author prefers intraoperative plain film radiographs to assess alignment better.

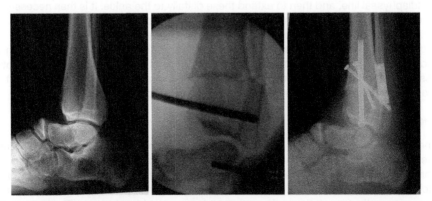

Fig. 8. Anterior ankle impingement resulting from clubfoot surgery. Hypoplastic talus and loss of height in the mortise lead to anterior plafond impingement. The patient was treated with FDO in the sagittal plane.

If there is residual translational deformity, the distal tibia can be translated to realign the talus beneath the tibial axis. Fixation can be delivered by means of a percutaneous method. In some circumstances, a medial plate can be used, but there is often a cortical stepoff at the level of the osteotomy that makes plating impractical.

An opening wedge osteotomy is planned and executed in the same way as the closing wedge osteotomy. Indications include osteotomy of the distal tibia requiring angulation and small amounts of length. This type of osteotomy is usually used to treat physeal disturbances and malunion resulting in varus deformity. There is little additional translation correction after the opening wedge is completed. The technique involves a linear incision over the base of the opening wedge. A guide wire is placed in the metaphyseal bone as an osteotomy guide. The periosteal sleeve is lifted in a circumferential fashion at the level of the osteotomy. The bone cut is made leaving a cortical hinge to improve stability,[8] and a Weinraub distractor or similar distractor is used to dial in the amount of desired correction. Intraoperative films verify the correction. Fixation is placed, and the void is filled with bone. The periosteal sleeve keeps the bone graft in place. Best and Daniels[18] described a technique with a platform (Puddu) plate placed inside the cortex of the osteotomy. Autogenous bone graft was used to fill the open wedge. Healing and incorporation of the graft were seen in all osteotomies at 12 weeks. A potential problem with opening wedge osteotomy is the tensioning of the medial soft tissues with varus correction. Sanders and colleagues[24] used neuromonitoring for any lengthening procedures to void iatrogenic nerve injury with deformity correction.

A modification of this technique involves a combined opening and closing wedge osteotomy (**Fig. 9**). This technique allows for maintenance of length while improving the degree of angular correction. The transverse nature of the closing wedge allows for additional translation with angulation correction.

TRIPLANE OSTEOTOMY

The triplane osteotomy (TO) is a technique that allows for deformity correction in all three planes. The osteotomy is based on the principle that any deformity has one axis of rotation around which the deformity can be corrected. Sangeorzan and colleagues[25] described a mathematic model for deformity planning and correction

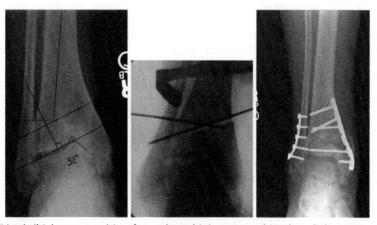

Fig. 9. Distal tibial varus resulting from physeal injury. A combined medial opening wedge and lateral closing wedge allows for correction near the CORA and maintains length.

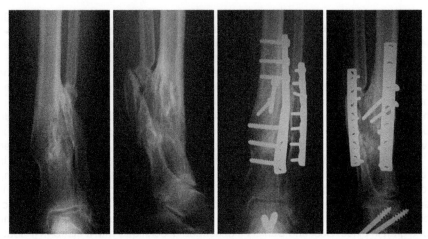

Fig. 10. Distal tibial malunion with valgus and recurvatum. The patient was treated with an oblique TO to correct valgus and recurvatum. Lateral tension plate fixation was used. A subtalar arthrodesis was required to realign the hind foot.

based on vector trigonometry. A carefully planned and executed osteotomy can realign the deformity in all three planes. The TO is ideally centered at the level of the CORA. The degree of correction in any plane is proportional to the amount of deviation from that plane. For example, a long oblique osteotomy made in the frontal plane affords frontal plane correction with little transverse or sagittal plane correction. In contrast an osteotomy of 45° with respect to all three planes affords equal correction in all three planes. This osteotomy is only useful for tibial malunion above the metaphysis. The author prefers fixation with lateral tension plating using standard internal fixation techniques (**Fig. 10**).

SUMMARY

SMO for posttraumatic malunion, developmental or physeal deformities, congenital malalignment, or focal articular degenerative problems in the ankle is a useful surgical technique. Accurate evaluation of the distal tibial deformity, weight-bearing radiographs, and soft tissue examination for contractures and instability ensure proper decision making. Osteotomy planning must involve all components of the deformity, including the foot, and respect osteotomy principles.

FURTHER READINGS

Stamatis ED, Cooper PS, Myerson MS. Supramalleolar osteotomy for the treatment of distal tibial angular deformities and arthritis of the ankle joint. Foot Ankle Int 2003; 24(10):754–64.

REFERENCES

1. Mendicino RW, Catanzariti AR, Reeves CL. Percutaneous supramalleolar osteotomy for distal tibial (near articular) ankle deformities. J Am Podiatr Med Assoc 2005;95(1):72–84.
2. Napiontek M, Nazar J. Tibial osteotomy as a salvage procedure in the treatment of congenital talipes equinovarus. J Pediatr Orthop 1994;14:763–7.

3. Abraham E, Lubicky JP, Songer MN. Supramalleolar osteotomy for ankle valgus in myelomeningocele. J Pediatr Orthop 1996;16:774–81.
4. Graehl PM, Hersh MR, Heckman JD. Supramalleolar osteotomy for the treatment of symptomatic tibial nonunion. J Orthop Trauma 1987;1:281–92.
5. McNicol D, Leong JC, Hsu LC. Supramalleolar derotation osteotomy for lateral tibial torsion and associated equinovarus deformity of the foot. J Bone Joint Surg Am 1983;65A:166–70.
6. Scheffer MM, Peterson HA. Opening-wedge osteotomy for angular deformities of long bones in children. J Bone Joint Surg Am 1994;76A:325–34.
7. Harstall R, Lehmann O, Krause F, et al. Supramalleolar lateral closing wedge osteotomy for the treatment of varus ankle arthrosis. Foot Ankle Int 2007;28(5): 542–8, 1994;76B:947–50.
8. Takakura Y, Takoaka T, Tanaka Y. Results of opening wedge osteotomy for the treatment of a post traumatic varus deformity of the ankle. J Bone Joint Surg Am 1998;80A:213–8.
9. Takakura Y, Tanaka Y, Kumai T. Low tibial osteotomy for osteoarthritis of the ankle. Results of a new operation in 18 patients. J Bone Joint Surg Am 1995;77B:50–4.
10. Heywood AW. Supramalleolar osteotomy in the management of the rheumatoid hindfoot. Clin Orthop 1983;177:76–81.
11. Pearce MS, Smith MA, Savidge GF. Supramalleolar tibial osteotomy for haemophilic arthropathy of the ankle. J Bone Joint Surg Am 1994;76B:947–50.
12. Merchant TC, Dietz FR. Long term follow up after fractures of the tibial and fibular shafts. J Bone Joint Surg Am 1989;71A:599–606.
13. Kristensen KD, Kiaer T, Blicher J. No arthrosis of the ankle 20 years after malaligned tibial shaft fracture. Acta Orthop Scand 1989;60:208–9.
14. Paley D. Ankle and foot considerations. In: Paley D, editor. Principles of deformity correction. New York: Springer; 2002. p. 46, 572, 573, 581.
15. Paley D. Normal limb alignment and joint orientation. In: Paley D, editor. Principles of deformity correction. New York: Springer; 2002.
16. Lamm BM, Paley D. Deformity correction planning for hindfoot, ankle, and lower limb. Clin Podiatr Med Surg 2004;21:305–26.
17. Ting AJ, Tarr RR, Sarmiento A. The role of subtalar motion and ankle contact pressure changes from angular deformities of the tibia. Foot Ankle 1987;7:290–9.
18. Best A, Daniels TR. Supramalleolar tibial osteotomy secured with the Puddu plate. Orthopedics 2006;29(6):537–40.
19. Tarr RR, Resnick CT, Wagner KS. Changes in tibiotalar joint contact areas following experimentally induced tibial angular deformities. Clin Orthop 1985;199:72–80.
20. Sammarco GJ. Biomechanics of the foot. In: Nordin M, Frankel VH, editors. Basic biomechanics of the musculoskeletal system. 2nd edition. Philadelphia: Lea & Febuger; 1989.
21. Inman VT. The joints of the ankle. Baltimore (MD): Williams and Wilkins; 1976.
22. Steffensmeier SJ, Saltzman CL, Berbaum KS. Effects of medial and lateral displacement calcaneal osteotomies on tibiotalar contact stresses. J Orthop Res 1996;14:980–5.
23. Paley D. Osteotomy concepts in frontal plane realignment. In: Paley D, editor. Principles of deformity correction. New York: Springer; 2002. p. 104.
24. Sanders R, Anglen JO, Mark JB. Oblique osteotomy for the correction of tibial malunion. J Bone Joint Surg Am 1995;77:240–6.
25. Sangeorzan BJ, Sangeorzan ST, Hansen ST Jr, et al. Mathematically directed single cut osteotomy for correction of tibial malunion. J Orthop Trauma 1989; 3(4):267–75.

Traditional Ankle Arthrodesis for the Treatment of Ankle Arthritis

Cody A. Bowers, DPM, Alan R. Catanzariti, DPM, FACFAS,
Robert W. Mendicino, DPM, FACFAS*

KEYWORDS

- Ankle arthritis • Degenerative joint disease of ankle
- Tibiotalar arthrodesis • Fusion of ankle

Ankle arthritis is a disabling condition that can cause significant pain and disability. The first reported technique for ankle arthrodesis in treating arthritis was published in 1879.[1] Early fusion rates, however, were low, and complication rates as high as 60% with nonunion rates of 40% have been reported.[2] There have been more than 40 different surgical techniques recommended for ankle arthrodesis.[3]

Improvements in operative technique and methods of fixation have led to significantly better rates of union and fewer complications. Studies by Kitaoka,[4] Mann and Rongstad,[5] and Morgan and colleagues[6] report approximately 90% union rates. The authors review the pathophysiology, diagnostic evaluation, treatment, and traditional methods of fixation for ankle arthrodesis.

ANATOMY

The ankle joint is composed of three articular surfaces: the medial articulation between the lateral tibial malleolus and the medial body of the talus, the lateral articulation between the medial fibular malleolus and lateral talar body, and the weight-bearing articulation of the talar dome and the distal tibial plafond. The ankle joint is a highly congruent joint with uniform cartilaginous surfaces. The thickness of the ankle cartilage ranges from 1.0 to 1.7 mm, significantly thinner than the 1.0- to 6.0-mm thick knee cartilage. Shepherd and Seedhom[7] studied the thickness of articular cartilage comparing the ankle, knee, and hip. They found an inverse relation between the thickness of the cartilage and its compression modulus. This evidence explains why the

---

Department of Foot and Ankle Surgery, The Western Pennsylvania Hospital, Pittsburgh, PA, USA
* Corresponding author. 4800 Friendship Avenue, N1, Pittsburgh, PA 15224.
E-mail address: rmendicino@faiwp.com (R. W. Mendicino).

Clin Podiatr Med Surg 26 (2009) 259–271
doi:10.1016/j.cpm.2008.12.003
0891-8422/08/$ – see front matter © 2009 Elsevier Inc. All rights reserved.

small surface area of the ankle joint is able to withstand large compressive weight-bearing forces with more resilience than the knee and hip joints.

The ankle joint is highly congruent; a wider talar dome anteriorly and more narrow in its posterior aspect creates a stable platform for the tibia in a static weight-bearing position. The total contact area of the ankle joint decreases by 13% to 18%, increasing the force per unit area when the foot is in a plantarflexed position.[8]

The most common cause of ankle arthritis is trauma. Pathologic conditions, such as malunited ankle fractures, cause significant change in the contact area of the tibiotalar articulation, and many studies have evaluated the congruency of an unstable or malaligned ankle.[9–11] The congruency of the ankle is directly affected by anatomic reduction of a fracture and the stability of the medial soft tissue structures. Malunited fibular fractures, untreated syndesmotic injuries, and compromise of the medial ankle support can all cause widening of the ankle mortise, allowing lateral shift of the talus within the joint. This can ultimately result in less total tibiotalar contact. Any malalignment of the fracture fragment within the ankle mortise also compromises the amount of surface area contact.

PATHOPHYSIOLOGY

Although posttraumatic arthritis is the most common cause of degenerative disease of the ankle, there are many other causes as well. Primary osteoarthritis does occur; however, the percentage of primary osteoarthritis causing degenerative joint disease is low. Chronic ankle instability; inflammatory diseases, such as rheumatoid arthritis; hemochromatosis; infection; neuropathic arthropathy; and tumor can also cause degenerative changes of the ankle joint.

Approximately 50% of ankle arthritis cases are a result of previous trauma. The type of fracture, degree of cartilage injury, and incongruity of the ankle joint are major contributing factors to the severity of the disease. In a study of 300 ankle fractures by Lindsjo,[12] the prevalence of posttraumatic arthritis was 14%, with 33% of all Weber C ankle fractures resulting in posttraumatic arthritis as compared with only 4% of Weber A ankle fractures. Lindsjo[12] also found that the presence of a posterior tibial fracture increased the prevalence of arthritis when compared with ankle fractures without a posterior fragment. Radiographic evidence of arthritis after an ankle fracture can be seen as soon as 2 years after the injury.

High-energy injuries resulting in pilon and talar fractures have a high incidence of posttraumatic arthritis. Avascular necrosis of the talus after fracture is reported to be a common contributing factor to ankle arthritis. This particular condition can be difficult to treat and requires debridement of nonviable bone to achieve appropriate bone-to-bone opposition.[4]

Chronic ankle instability with recurrent ankle sprains can cause osteochondral lesions of the talar dome. Anterior subluxation and talar tilt within the ankle mortise cause significant changes in the tibiotalar contact area and are common causes of degenerative disease of the ankle in conjunction with instability.

Inflammatory diseases cause thickening of the ankle synovium, osseous erosion, and osteopenia. Diseases like rheumatoid arthritis, psoriatic arthritis, Reiter's syndrome, and ankylosing spondylitis can all lead to ankle arthritis. Arthritis of other joints of the foot in addition to the ankle and bilateral symptoms are common with inflammatory disease. Hemochromatosis and infection can lead to cartilage damage and destruction. Chronic inflammatory changes from these conditions can lead to joint changes.

DIAGNOSIS

The primary presenting symptom for a patient who has ankle arthritis is pain. A complete and thorough history should be obtained with emphasis on previous trauma, infection, systemic diseases, and previous treatment. Anti-inflammatory medication, orthotics, bracing, and physical therapy are all first-line treatment options that may have been initiated by the primary care or referring physician. The patient's social history, including use of tobacco, alcohol, and occupation, should be considered when formulating a treatment plan. A study by Cobb and colleagues[13] reported that smokers had a 16-fold increased risk for nonunion compared with nonsmokers.

The physical examination should be comprehensive as well. Incision sites from previous surgery and the presence of atrophic skin near the proposed incision site should be noted. Open ulcerations or wound dehiscence should be treated before surgical intervention. Maximum points of tenderness should be noted on all aspects of the ankle and correlated to anatomic structures. Vascular examination should include palpation of pulses, presence of edema, and pedal hair growth. If pulses are not palpable, noninvasive vascular testing is recommended before surgical intervention. The alignment and mobility of the foot and ankle should be evaluated weight bearing and non-weight bearing, because frontal plane deformity of the rearfoot might alter the operative plan. Limitation in dorsiflexion of the ankle joint signifies equinus deformity and may need to be addressed by performing a posterior muscle group lengthening to enable the surgeon to realign the ankle. Monofilament sensory testing is important to evaluate for neurologic deficits.

Radiographic analysis includes weight-bearing films of the foot and ankle. Anteroposterior, mortise, and lateral views of the ankle should be obtained in addition to anteroposterior and medial oblique views of the foot. Joint space, alignment, presence and location of osteophytes, and osteopenia should all be noted (**Fig. 1**). Fibular length is often compromised in the posttraumatic patient who has ankle arthritis. In cases of

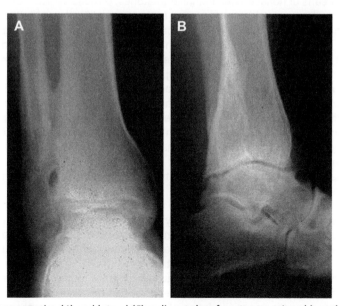

Fig. 1. Anteroposterior (A) and lateral (B) radiographs of posttraumatic ankle arthritis. Note the joint space narrowing, sclerotic bone, and osteophytes.

severe deformity, hind foot realignment and long leg calcaneal axial projections should be obtained to evaluate lower leg, ankle, and foot alignment further.[14]

Further imaging studies, including MRI and CT, may be beneficial to rule out avascular bone or assess surrounding soft tissue structures. MRI can reveal the integrity of cartilaginous surfaces or presence of infection if that is suspected. CT scans enable the physician to evaluate osseous healing of previous fractures and pathologic findings in adjacent joints. This can be particularly helpful when the quality of the subtalar joint is also in question. Although advanced imaging is not routinely ordered, it can provide diagnostic information and aid preoperative planning.

Intra-articular injections can be diagnostic and therapeutic. These can be used for nonoperative treatment of degenerative ankle disease. An injection of corticosteroid is used to decrease inflammation and pain within the joint. Although there are no studies that demonstrate the effects of corticosteroid injection in the arthritic ankle, there are numerous studies documenting its success for the knee joint.[15–17] Combining the corticosteroid with a local anesthetic enables the physician to ascertain what structures might be contributing to the patient's symptom complex. Injecting the ankle with local anesthetic and obtaining 100% pain relief assures the physician that the ankle is the only joint involved. A physical examination that elicits point tenderness in the sinus tarsi might raise suspicion that the subtalar joint is also affected. A second injection in the subtalar joint can help to diagnose subtalar joint degenerative disease. The surgical treatment may then include fusion of the subtalar joint. It is also important to determine if the patient's pain is completely osseous in nature, because many conditions have associated malalignment and may be causing soft tissue impingement and tendinous pathologic changes.

TREATMENT

Primary nonoperative care for ankle arthritis is focused on decreasing pain and inflammation by means of nonsteroidal anti-inflammatories, orthotic devices, braces, corticosteroid injections, physical therapy, and foot gear modifications. Modification and termination of those activities that cause pain can help to alleviate symptoms if the patient has a high body mass index. Weight loss programs might lead to decreased pain in the lower extremity joints. Assistive devices, such as a cane, can be used for stability and to decrease weight bearing.

Many bracing modalities can be prescribed to decrease ankle motion and to offload the ankle joint. Adding a rocker to the plantar surface of shoes decreases the need for ankle dorsiflexion during normal gait. Lace-up ankle braces provide support to an unstable ankle joint and may alleviate pain in a mildly arthritic joint. Custom ankle-foot orthoses may also alleviate symptoms by supporting the ankle and hind foot joints, in addition to decreasing motion. Offloading braces, such as a patellar tendon–bearing brace, are useful in patients who have more advanced arthritis and may not be surgical candidates.

Ankle arthrocentesis may be effective in decreasing the pain and inflammation of a degenerated ankle joint. Pain relief may range from complete to minimal relief, with the duration of relief experienced being variable. It is important for patients to relate to the physician how much relief was obtained and how long the pain relief lasted after receiving a corticosteroid injection.

Various types of surgical therapy are available for ankle arthritis. Surgical debridement of degenerative bone, open or arthroscopic, can be beneficial in a patient with relatively good cartilaginous surfaces. Debriding periarticular osteophytes can produce good results if the cartilage of the talus and tibia is minimally affected.

Patients who respond best to this treatment have a relatively good joint space, with impinging synovium or loose bodies within the ankle joint. Chondral lesions less than 1 cm in diameter may respond well to debridement with subchondral drilling and microfracture.

More recently, attention has been directed toward arthroscopically treated ankle arthritis. This provides an excellent alternative to open debridement because of its limited soft tissue dissection and decreased convalescence. This is discussed in detail in other articles in this issue. In general, arthroscopic debridement has not proved effective in the severely arthritic joint with joint space narrowing.

ANKLE ARTHRODESIS TECHNIQUE

The "gold standard" for treatment of severe ankle arthritis is arthrodesis, and the primary indication for this procedure is debilitating arthritic ankle pain limiting daily activity. The patient should be educated, and patient expectations should be clearly discussed before surgery. The patient should be aware of potential complications, including infection, nonunion or delayed union, neurologic deficits, and the possibility of needing revisional surgery if primary arthrodesis fails. The potential for limb shortening, prolonged immobilization, need for external fixation, use of biologic materials, and shoe modifications should all be understood by the patient before surgical intervention.

The surgery involves spinal or general anesthetic. The authors position the patient in the supine position with a bump under the ipsilateral hip so that the patella is in a forward position. After appropriate positioning of the knee, the surgical leg is placed on a raised platform to ensure access to the medial and lateral ankle and to prevent the contralateral limb from interfering with laterally projected fluoroscopic images. A pneumatic thigh tourniquet is used for hemostasis. Surgical preparation up to the level of the knee is performed to enable the surgeons to visualize the entire lower leg during surgery.

The traditional method of performing arthrodesis of the tibiotalar joint involves a two-incision approach. The lateral incision is placed directly lateral over the fibula beginning 7 cm proximal to the tibial plafond and extending 1 cm distal to the tip of the fibular malleolus (**Fig. 2**). The incision is carried through skin and subcutaneous tissues. Care should be taken to preserve all neurovascular structures, keeping in mind normal variants in the course of the sural nerve and the location of the perforating peroneal artery. The periosteum of the fibula is incised in a linear fashion, and all soft tissue attachments are released. The fibula is transected on an oblique plane from proximal-lateral to distal-medial beginning approximately 1.5 cm proximal to the tibial plafond (**Fig. 3**). The distal portion of fibula is then removed from the surgical site and kept sterile on the back table for use as a structural or morselized bone graft (**Fig. 4**). The soft tissue and ankle capsule of the anterior tibia are released, creating a plane across the anterior ankle joint deep to all vital neurovascular structures.

A linear medial incision is made overlying the medial gutter (**Fig. 5**). The saphenous nerve and vein should be identified in this area and preserved. Soft tissues are then released from the adjacent areas of the tibia and talus to expose the tibia, talus, and medial gutter (**Fig. 6**). A malleable retractor is then bent in a U-shape and placed deep to the soft tissues to provide appropriate retraction of the anterior neurovascular and tendinous structures (**Fig. 7**). The area is now prepared for resection of the articular surfaces.

The surgeon can use fluoroscopy to determine the appropriate position of the osseous cuts. Surgeons may also place Kirschner wires as axis guides to ensure

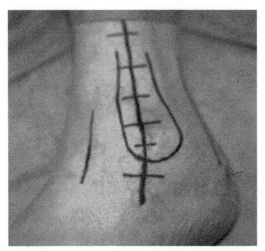

Fig. 2. The lateral incision is directly over the fibula and long enough to expose the surgical site adequately.

proper planar resection of the articular surfaces. Either method is appropriate, but it is paramount that any osseous deformity within the joint is corrected during planar resection. This ensures the desired position during fusion. The first cut is a notch made anterior to posterior within the medial malleolus. The blade is released from the saw and left in place to protect the medial malleolus from being osteotomized (**Fig. 8**). With a second blade attached to the saw, the tibial cartilage is resected from lateral to medial under image intensification (**Fig. 9**). Under this projection, the

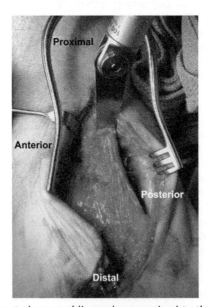

Fig. 3. The fibula is transected on an oblique plane proximal to the ankle joint.

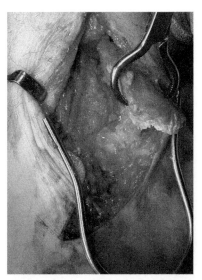

Fig. 4. The distal portion of the fibula is resected and used for on-lay graft or morselized for autogenous bone graft.

surgeon can be certain that the cut is planar in the coronal and sagittal planes. The saw blade remaining in the medial gutter prevents overextending the saw and transecting the medial malleolus.

The foot is then placed in the appropriate position: neutral dorsiflexion, slight valgus, and 5° of abduction.[18] The position is confirmed under fluoroscopy. The talus should be translated slightly posterior to shorten the foot and lever arm (**Fig. 10**). Approximately 3 to 5 mm of the talar dome is resected to expose the cancellous bone of the talar body (**Fig. 11**). The subchondral plates are then drilled with a Kirschner

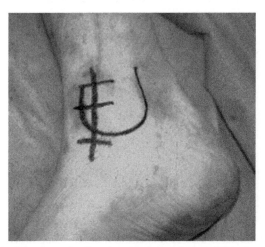

Fig. 5. The second incision is made directly anterior to the medial gutter.

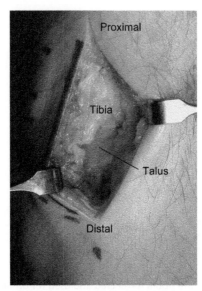

Fig. 6. The soft tissues are reflected, exposing the tibia, talus, and medial gutter.

wire or fish-scaled using a small osteotome, preparing the joint surfaces for arthrodesis.

Glissan's[19] principles of arthrodesis should be followed whenever an arthrodesing procedure is performed:

- Adequate joint debridement and preparation
- Accurate coaptation of surfaces
- Optimal position
- Maintain position until arthrodesis is sound

The foot is placed in its optimal position (**Fig. 12**), and guide pins are placed for provisional fixation. The placement of fixation can be performed with cannulated or

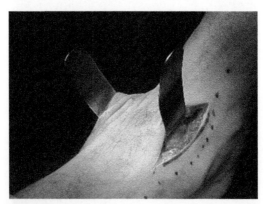

Fig. 7. A malleable retractor is used to retract the vital soft tissue structures in the anterior ankle in preparation for joint resection.

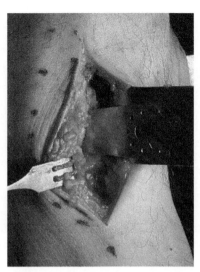

Fig. 8. The saw blade is left in the medial gutter to prevent transecting of the tibial malleolus during joint resection.

noncannulated screws, consistent with AO fixation principles. The first point of fixation is placed from the lateral talar process, crossing the ankle joint, aiming at the medial shoulder of the tibia. The second point of fixation should be placed from the medial malleolus, grasping the talar body parallel to the first screw. The third point of fixation begins in the anterolateral tibia at the level of the transected fibular and crosses the joint running medially and slightly posterior into the body of the talus. Appropriate length partially threaded screws are then placed over the guide pins for fixation. Osteosynthesis is performed with image intensification.

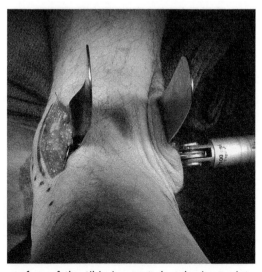

Fig. 9. The articular surface of the tibia is resected under image intensification ensuring appropriate positioning in all planes.

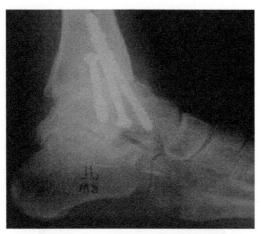

Fig. 10. Inappropriate positioning of the talus under the tibia can result in foot forwardus and an undesirable result.

Clinical positioning of the foot should be confirmed after removal of all guide pins. Final anteroposterior and lateral radiographs should illustrate osseous coaptation of the tibia and talus, proper positioning in all planes, and a rigid fixation construct. The three points of fixation provide stability and compressive forces across the ankle joint (**Fig. 13**). If three screws are not possible, a construct of two crossing screws is also acceptable.

The surgical incisions are closed in layers after copious sterile saline lavage. The ankle capsule should be closed with 2-0 absorbable suture. The skin edges are

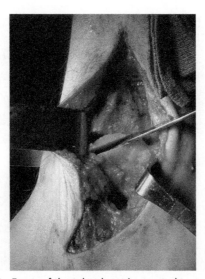

Fig. 11. Approximately 3 to 5 mm of the talar dome is resected to reveal cancellous bone and provide a stable surface for arthrodesis.

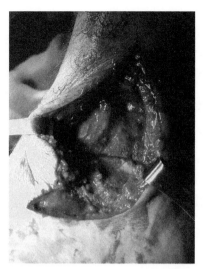

Fig. 12. The tibia and talus are optimally positioned under image intensification and temporarily fixated.

then brought together with subcutaneous 3-0 or 4-0 absorbable sutures, followed by skin closure with nonabsorbable suture or skin staples (**Fig. 14**).

The patient is placed in a compressive dressing and a posterior fiberglass splint. The primary surgeon commonly admits the patient to the hospital for 23-hour observation and pain control. The dressings are removed on postoperative day 1 if pain is well controlled, the operative site is inspected, and the patient is placed in a short-leg fiberglass cast. Sutures can be removed at 2 weeks. Partial weight bearing is initiated at 6 to 8 weeks based on serial radiographs. Protected weight bearing is instituted for an additional 4 to 6 weeks. Serial radiographs are used to evaluate the arthrodesis site throughout the postoperative period.

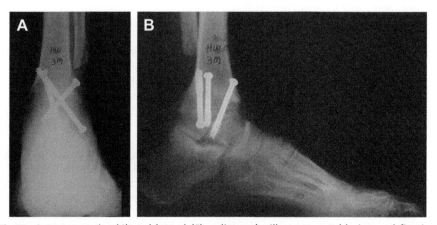

Fig. 13. Anteroposterior (*A*) and lateral (*B*) radiographs illustrate a stable internal fixation construct and optimal positioning.

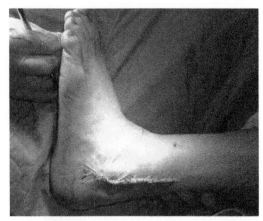

Fig. 14. Postoperative clinical picture after skin closure demonstrates the foot at 90° to the leg in the sagittal plane.

SUMMARY

Ankle arthrodesis has proved to be a reasonable surgical intervention for degenerative joint disease when nonoperative measures have failed. Numerous studies have provided evidence that traditional ankle fusion with internal fixation provides a high success rate.[20–24] The outcomes are enhanced with adequate joint preparation, proper alignment, a stiff fixation construct, and long-term immobilization.

REFERENCES

1. Aaron AD. Ankle fusion: a retrospective review. Orthopedics 1990;13:1249–54.
2. Raikin SM. Arthrodesis of the ankle: arthroscopic, mini-open, and open techniques. Foot Ankle Clin 2003;8:347–59.
3. Vogler H. Ankle arthrodesis: clinical and conceptual applications. Clin Podiatry 1985;2:59–80.
4. Kitaoka HB. Arthrodesis of the ankle: technique, complications, and salvage treatment. Instr Course Lect 1999;48:255–61.
5. Mann RA, Rongstad KM. Arthrodesis of the ankle: a critical analysis. Foot Ankle Int 1998;19:3–9.
6. Morgan CD, Henki JA, Bailey RW, et al. Long-term results of tibiotalar arthrodesis. J Bone Joint Surg Am 1985;67:546–9.
7. Shepherd DE, Seedhom BB. Thickness of human articular cartilage in joints of the lower limb. Ann Rheum Dis 1999;58:27–34.
8. Calhoun JH, Li F, Ledbetter BR, et al. A comprehensive study of pressure distribution in the ankle joint with inversion and eversion. Foot Ankle Int 1994;15:125–33.
9. Clark HJ, Michelson JK, Cox QG, et al. Tibio-talar stability in bimalleolar ankle fractures: a dynamic in vitro contact area study. Foot Ankle 1991;11:222–7.
10. Pereira DS, Koval KJ, Resnick RB, et al. Tibiotalar contact area and pressure distribution: the effect of mortise widening and syndesmosis fixation. Foot Ankle Int 1996;17:269–74.
11. Ramsey PL, Hamilton W. Changes in tibiotalar area of contact caused by lateral talar shift. J Bone Joint Surg Am 1976;58:356–7.

12. Lindsjo U. Operative treatment of ankle fracture-dislocations. A follow-up study of 306/321 consecutive cases. Clin Orthop 1985;199:28–38.

13. Cobb TK, Gabrielsen TA, Campbell DC 2nd, et al. Cigarette smoking and nonunion after ankle arthrodesis. Foot Ankle Int 1994;15:64–7.

14. Mendicino RW, Catanzariti AR, John John S, et al. Long leg calcaneal axial and hindfoot alignment radiographic views for frontal plane assessment. J Am Podiatr Med Assoc 2008;98:75–8.

15. Friedman DM, Moore ME. The efficacy of intraarticular steroids in osteoarthritis: a double-blind study. J Rheumatol 1980;7:850–6.

16. Gaffney K, Ledingham J, Perry JD. Intra-articular triamcinolone hexacetonide in knee osteoarthritis: factors influencing the clinical response. Ann Rheum Dis 1995;54:379–81.

17. Jones A, Doherty M. Intra-articular corticosteroids are effective in osteoarthritis but there are no clinical predictors of response. Ann Rheum Dis 1996;55:829–32.

18. Mendicino RW, Lamm BM, Catanzariti AR, et al. Realignment arthrodesis of the rearfoot and ankle: a comprehensive evaluation. J Am Podiatr Med Assoc 2005;95(1):60–71.

19. Glissan DJ. The indications for inducing fusion at the ankle joint by operation with description of two successful techniques. Aust N Z J Surg 1949;19:64–71.

20. Chen YJ, Huang TJ, Shih HN, et al. Ankle arthrodesis with cross screw fixation. Good results in 36/40 cases followed 3–7 years. Acta Orthop Scand 1996;67: 473–8.

21. Coester LM, Saltzman CL, Leupold J, et al. Long-term results following ankle arthrodesis for post-traumatic arthritis. J Bone Joint Surg Am 2001;83(2):219–28.

22. Colman AB, Pomeroy GC. Transfibular ankle arthrodesis with rigid internal fixation: an assessment of outcome. Foot Ankle Int 2007;28:303–7.

23. Mahan KT, Yu G, Kalish SR. Podiatry Institute ankle fusion technique. J Am Podiatr Med Assoc 1997;87:101–16.

24. Thomas RH, Daniels TR. Current concepts review: ankle arthritis. J Bone Joint Surg Am 2003;85(5):923–36.

Arthroscopic Ankle Arthrodesis

Michael S. Lee, DPM, FACFAS[a,b,*], David M. Millward, BS[a]

KEYWORDS

- Ankle • Arthrodesis • Arthroscopy • Fusion • Arthritis

Despite the increasing popularity of total ankle replacement (TAR), ankle arthrodesis remains the gold standard for the treatment of end-stage ankle arthritis.[1,2] Historically, open techniques have been used for ankle arthrodesis. There have been many variations and techniques described including transfibular, anterior, medial, and miniarthrotomy.[3–17] Inherent disadvantages to these open techniques include postoperative pain, delayed union or nonunion, wound complications, shortening, prolonged healing times, and prolonged hospital stays.[18–20]

Arthroscopic ankle arthrodesis provides the foot and ankle surgeon with an alternative to the traditional open techniques. Arthroscopic ankle arthrodesis has demonstrated faster union rates, decreased complications, reduced postoperative pain, and shorter hospital stays.[3,20–29] Once considered technically difficult, advancements in techniques and instrumentation have decreased the learning curve formerly encountered with the arthroscopic technique.

Schneider[30] investigated arthroscopic ankle arthrodesis in 1983 and reported faster time to union, earlier mobilization, and reduced patient morbidity. More recent studies have demonstrated similar results with faster union rates, fewer complications, shorter hospital stays with union rates comparable to more recent open techniques. This article explores the indications, technique, and complications associated with arthroscopic ankle arthrodesis.

INDICATIONS AND CONTRAINDICATIONS

Arthroscopic ankle arthrodesis may be indicated in patients with end-stage arthritis due to a variety of causes including: rheumatoid arthritis, posttraumatic arthritis, arthrogryposis, septic arthritis, inflammatory arthritis, avascular necrosis of the talus, idiopathic osteoarthritis, chronic ankle instability secondary to polio, and (the most frequently encountered) posttraumatic arthritis.[21]

---

[a] College of Podiatric Medicine and Surgery, Des Moines University, Des Moines, IA, USA
[b] Foot and Ankle Surgery, Capital Orthopaedics and Sports Medicine, 1601 NW 114th Street, Suite 142, Des Moines, IA 50325, USA
* Corresponding author. College of Podiatric Medicine and Surgery, Des Moines University, Des Moines, Iowa.
E-mail address: mlee@dsmcapitalortho.com (M.S. Lee).

Clin Podiatr Med Surg 26 (2009) 273–282
doi:10.1016/j.cpm.2009.03.002
0891-8422/09/$ – see front matter © 2009 Elsevier Inc. All rights reserved.

The primary indication for ankle arthrodesis is persistent pain in the arthritic ankle joint that has not responded to conservative treatments including analgesics, nonsteroidal anti-inflammatory drugs, corticosteroid injections, orthoses, or bracing for 6 or more months.[3,22,28] While not currently US Federal Drug Administration approved for the ankle joint, hyaluronase injections are also often used by the senior author before proceeding with arthrodesis or replacement.

Limitations of arthroscopic ankle arthrodesis are typically related to deformity or malalignment about the ankle joint. Various studies have indicated that malalignment greater than 10 to 15 degrees will make reduction of the ankle joint and deformity difficult.[23,31] Ferkel and Hewitt[27] indicated that patients with significant ankle deformity, of either significant varus or valgus, are better suited for an open technique and those that require arthrodesis in situ are better suited for the arthroscopic technique. Tang and colleagues[32] stated that arthroscopy should not be advised when a large ankle deformity is present. A study done in 2007 by Gougoulias and colleagues[26] showed that patients with marked deformity of greater than 10 to 15 degrees of varus or valgus can be treated effectively using arthroscopy, depending on the surgeon's experience.

In addition to significant malalignment, Collman and colleagues[22] noted that contraindications of arthroscopic ankle arthrodesis include excessive bone loss, neuropathic joints, active infections, and poor bone stock. Avascular necrosis of the talus may also be contraindication.

SURGICAL TECHNIQUE

Arthroscopic ankle arthrodesis is performed under general or spinal anesthesia. A thigh tourniquet is used for hemostasis and the leg is typically prepped to the tibial tuberosity. A bump under the ipsilateral hip is used internally to rotate the leg to place the malleoli in the frontal plane.

The ankle is insufflated with approximately 20-mL of normal sterile saline (NSS) using an 18-gauge needle. Standard anteromedial and anterolateral portals are used. A 2.7 millimeter (mm), 30° arthroscope is then introduced into the ankle joint. The senior author prefers to use large joint power shavers and burrs while using a 2.7 mm arthroscope rather than the 4.0 mm arthroscope. A noninvasive ankle distractor is applied to the ankle to allow for complete visualization from anterior to posterior, as well as both the medial and lateral gutters (**Fig. 1**).

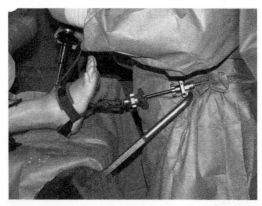

Fig. 1. Noninvasive ankle distractor being used for joint visualization.

A 3.85 mm full radius incisor blade is used to aggressively debride the anterior joint of any hypertrophic synovium, fibrosis, or loose bodies. In some cases, aggressive resection of anterior tibiotalar osteophytes is required for proper joint visualization. A curette is inserted to aggressively remove any articular cartilage (**Fig. 2**). A grasping forceps or resector may be used to remove the cartilage fragments (**Fig. 3**). A 4.0 mm full radius burr or 4.85 mm burr is then used to resect the subchondral plate (**Fig. 4**). A curved osteotome is then used to further fish scale the subchondral plates of the tibia and talus (**Fig. 5**). Ideally, healthy bleeding bone will be visualized throughout the tibiotalar articulation (**Fig. 6**). The joint is then irrigated and all loose bodies or fragments are evacuated.

All arthroscopic instrumentation is then removed from the ankle joint. Platelet-rich plasma or other bone graft substitutes may then be inserted into the ankle joint. The noninvasive distraction is removed from the foot. Proper bony apposition is confirmed using fluoroscopy. Care is also taken to confirm proper positioning both clinically and radiographically.

Fixation is typically achieved with two or three large diameter cannulated screws. One is placed from the lateral talar process into the medial tibia, the second from the posterior tibia into the talar neck, and the third (if desired) from the lateral tibia into the posteromedial talus (**Fig. 7**).

The portals and stab incisions for screw placement are closed with simple sutures. The extremity is placed in an immobilizer boot. In most cases, the patient is discharged to home the day of surgery. Sutures are removed at 1 week after the operation and the patient is placed in a below-the-knee cast. Strict adherence to non-weight bearing is followed for 6 to 7 weeks. Weight bearing is then advanced based on radiographic healing and clinical symptoms in an immobilizer boot (**Fig. 8**). Typically, at approximately 10 weeks after the operation, the patient is placed in a rocker-bottom sole shoe and ankle-foot-orthoses (AFO), and activities are advanced as tolerated. Use of the AFO is continued for up to an additional 3 months and the rocker-bottom sole is continued according to the patient's preference.

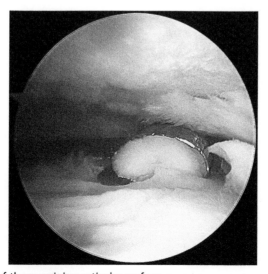

Fig. 2. Curettage of the remaining articular surface.

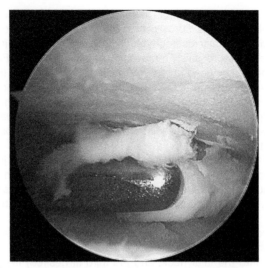

Fig. 3. Removal of the cartilage fragments after aggressive curettage.

DISCUSSION

Arthroscopic ankle arthrodesis has been well studied and has demonstrated favorable postoperative outcomes.[20–29] Advantages include decreased time to union, diminished postoperative pain, comparable union rates, shorter hospital stays, and earlier patient mobilization.[20–29,33–36] Preservation of the bony contour and the large amount of cancellous bone contact allows for significant stability and rigid internal fixation.[22,36] This is contradictory to the traditional open techniques which have often implemented planal resection decreasing bony contact and decreasing inherent stability. Additionally, "flat-topping" the talus and tibia makes proper positioning of the foot in the

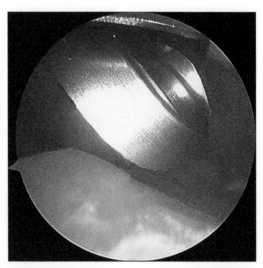

Fig. 4. Full radius burr being used to resect the subchondral plate.

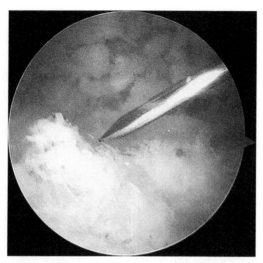

Fig. 5. Fish scaling the talus with a curved osteotome in preparation for arthrodesis.

sagittal plane significantly more difficult, as precise bone cuts are required. O'Brien and colleagues[20] showed there was greater variability of ankle positions in patients that received the open ankle fusion compared with the arthroscopic technique.

Stetson and Ferkel[31] recommended an open technique in ankles that have malrotation or anterior-posterior translation of the tibiotalar joint. They also believed ankles that had a deformity of greater than 15 degrees of varus or valgus should be treated with an open technique. Gougoulias and colleagues,[26] however, achieved successful arthroscopic ankle arthrodeses on ankle deformities of 15 to 45 degrees of varus or valgus. They point out that, although they were able to successfully fuse ankles with marked deformity, there is a significant learning curve associated with the procedure.[26] Another recent study also suggests that it may be possible to fuse ankles

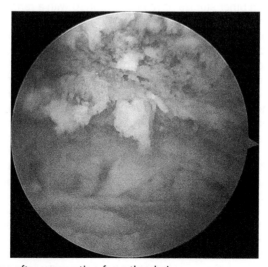

Fig. 6. Joint surfaces after preparation for arthrodesis.

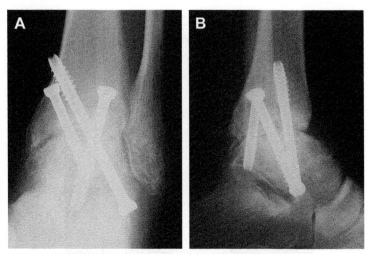

Fig. 7. (*A, B*) Typical fixation after arthroscopic ankle arthrodesis.

with deformities of 25 degrees or greater arthroscopically.[23] The senior author has found that malalignment up to 15 degrees is acceptable for arthroscopic arthrodesis. In some case, particularly in severe valgus malalignment of the ankle, the joint is reducible clinically. In these cases, arthroscopic ankle arthrodesis is possible but preoperative planning includes the possibility of converting to a miniarthrotomy.

Union may be described in two different ways: clinical union and radiographic union. Clinical union is described as having a stable, painless ankle joint. Radiographic union is defined as having bridging trabeculae between the tibia and the talus.[26,37]

Interestingly, nonunion rates between arthroscopic ankle arthrodesis and open techniques are similar. Crosby and colleagues[38] reported a 93% clinical fusion rate and a 74% radiographic union rate, indicating a subset of arthroscopic ankle arthrodesis cases that have clinical union rate of 87.2%. A nonunion rate of 7.6% was reported by Winson and colleagues[23] in their review of 118 arthroscopic ankle fusions. Similar union rates in other studies have been reported with a range from 73% up to 100%.[3,17,20,27–29,33,35,38–40]

Studies demonstrating union rates correlated to patient comorbidities have been limited primarily to rheumatoid arthritis.[39,41,42] Other variables such as history of smoking, arthritis etiology, effects of bone graft substitutes, body mass index, and pre-existing deformity have not been extensively studied with regard to arthroscopic ankle arthrodesis. In one study, four of five reported nonunions were in patients with posttraumatic arthritis.[22] The higher concentration of sclerotic bone adjacent to the subchondral plate may contribute to this increased incidence of nonunion, reinforcing the importance of aggressive joint resection.[29,33,41,43] Malalignment of the ankle may also predispose to nonunion of the arthroscopic ankle arthrodesis.[22]

Cigarette smoking and its negative effects on both soft-tissue and bone healing has been well documented.[44–49] The role of nicotine in ankle arthrodesis nonunions has also been well documented, and may present a relative risk of nonunion four times that seen in nonsmokers.[18,50] Collman and colleagues[22] did not see this same trend in their series of arthroscopic ankle fusions and theorized that the ill-effects of smoking are countered by the minimally invasive approach.

A clear advantage to the use of arthroscopic arthrodesis over open techniques is the time to fusion is reduced. Open ankle fusions have a reported average fusion time of

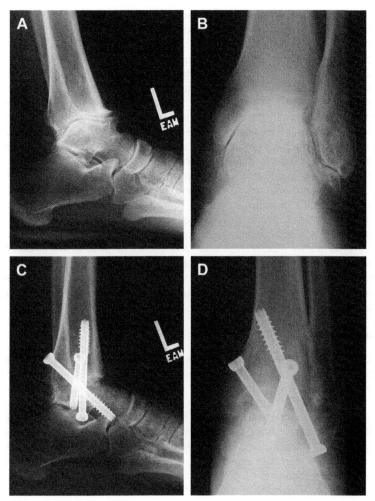

Fig. 8. (A, B, C, D) Preoperative and postoperative radiographs for arthroscopic ankle arthrodesis.

approximately 14 weeks.[33,34] In a study of 39 arthroscopic arthrodeses, Collman and colleagues[22] reported an average fusion time of 47 days, while Glick and colleagues[35] noted a 9-week average fusion time in 34 ankles. Other studies have noted time to fusion for arthroscopic ankle arthrodesis from 8.9 to 12 weeks.[3,23,29] One theory to support the decreased fusion time is that the arthroscopic technique does not disrupt the periarticular blood supply facilitating healing.[29,33,35,41]

O'Brien demonstrated that the tourniquet time, blood loss, and hospitalization time where all decreased using arthroscopy.[20] Patients who underwent arthroscopic arthrodesis had hospital stays of 1.6 days, versus the open techniques that averaged 3.4 days in the hospital.[20] Use of the arthroscopic technique may greatly reduce the postoperative hospitalization period. Ogilvie-Harris and colleagues[28] reported an average discharge from the hospital of 1 day. Dent and colleagues[25] also report an average stay of less than 2 days. Zvijac and colleagues[29] reported an average hospitalization of 3 days for those who had an open procedure as compared with 1 day for those who received an arthroscopic arthrodesis. They noted pain levels where much less than expected in the arthroscopic group. This lead them to perform arthroscopic ankle arthrodesis on an outpatient basis.[29] Cameron and Ulrich[3] also reported doing arthroscopic ankle arthrodesis as an outpatient procedure. In another study of 39 patients, only 3 were not discharged the day of the procedure.[22] Arthroscopic ankle arthrodesis has demonstrated reduced pain postoperatively and a shorter reliance on pain medication.[25,28,29] The senior author has also noted a significant decrease in postoperative pain with the arthroscopic technique. It is now common practice for arthroscopic ankle arthrodeses to be performed in outpatient surgery centers and, generally, the decision to admit a patient postoperatively is based on comorbid deformities and not postoperative-pain concerns.

Other advantages of arthroscopic arthrodesis include decreased blood loss, less disruption of the soft tissue structures around the ankle, and diminished risk of thrombosis due to shorter immobilization times. There is also minimal loss of length of the lower limb, and minimal clinical deformity or shape-changes to the ankle.[25]

Arthroscopic ankle arthrodesis may be preferred to an open technique in at-risk patients.[22] The earlier mobilization due to a shorter time to union is beneficial in patients with rheumatoid arthritis, advanced age, diabetes, and other autoimmune diseases.[33,40] The senior author has used the arthroscopic technique in these at-risk patients with great success, but cautions its use in patients with peripheral neuropathy.

SUMMARY

Arthroscopic ankle arthrodesis provides the foot and ankle surgeon with an alternative to traditional open techniques. Advancements in arthroscopic techniques and instrumentation have made the procedure easier to perform. Arthroscopic ankle arthrodesis has demonstrated faster rates of union, decreased complications, reduced postoperative pain, and shorter hospital stays.[3,20–29] Adherence to sound surgical techniques, particularly with regards to joint preparation is critical for success. Comorbidities such as increased body mass index, history of smoking, malalignment, and posttraumatic arthritis should be carefully considered when contemplating arthroscopic ankle arthrodesis. While total ankle replacement continues to grow in popularity, arthroscopic ankle arthrodesis remains a viable alternative for management of the end-stage arthritic ankle.

REFERENCES

1. Coester LM, Saltman CL, Leapold J, et al. Long-term results following ankle arthrodesis for post-traumatic arthritis. J Bone Joint Surg Am 2001;83:219–28.
2. Buck P, Morrey BF, Chao EY. The optimum position of arthrodesis of the ankle. J Bone Joint Surg Am 1987;69:1052–62.
3. Cameron SE, Ulrich P. Arthroscopic arthrodesis of the ankle joint. Arthroscopy 2000;16:21–6.
4. Cheng YM, Chen SK, Chen JC, et al. Revision of ankle arthrodesis. Foot Ankle Int 2003;24:321–5.
5. Colgrove RC, Bruffey JD. Ankle arthrodesis: combined internal-external fixation. Foot Ankle Int 2001;22:92–7.
6. Adams JC. Arthrodesis of the ankle joint: experiences with transfibular approach. J Bone Joint Surg Am 1948;30(B):506–11.
7. Frankel JP, Bacardi BE. Chevron ankle arthrodesis with bone grafting and internal fixation. J Foot Surg 1986;25:234–40.

8. Anderson R. Concentric arthrodesis of the ankle joint: a transmalleolar approach. J Bone Joint Surg 1945;27:37–48.
9. Baciu CC. A simple technique for arthrodesis of the ankle. J Bone Joint Surg Br 1986;68(2):266–7.
10. Campbell P. Arthrodesis of the ankle with modified distraction-compression and bone-grafting. J Bone Joint Surg 1990;72:552–6.
11. Campbell CJ, Rinehart WT, Kalenak A. Arthrodesis of the ankle: deep autogenous inlay grafts with maximum cancellous bone apposition. J Bone Joint Surg 1974; 56:63–70.
12. Vogler HW. Ankle fusion: techniques and complications. J Foot Surg 1991;30: 80–4.
13. Thordarson DB, Markolf KL, Cracchiolo A. Arthrodesis of the ankle with cancellous-bone screws and fibular strut graft. Biomechanical analysis. J Bone Joint Surg 1990;72:1359–63.
14. Mauerer RC, Cimino WR, Cox CV, et al. Transarticular cross-screw fixation; a technique of ankle arthrodesis. Clin Orthop 1991;268:56–69.
15. Morgan CD, Henke JA, Bailey RW, et al. Long-term results of tibiotalar arthrodesis. J Bone Joint Surg 1985;67:546–50.
16. Mears DC, Gordon RG, Kann SE, et al. Ankle arthrodesis with an anterior tension plate. Clin Orthop 1991;268:70–7.
17. Paremain GD, Miller SD, Myerson MS. Ankle arthrodesis: results after the miniarthrotomy technique. Foot Ankle Int 1996;17:247–51.
18. Frey C, Halikus NM, Vu-Rose T, et al. A review of ankle arthrodesis: predisposing factors to nonunion. Foot Ankle Int 1994;15(11):581–4.
19. Morrey BF, Wiedeman GP Jr. Complications and long-term results of ankle arthrodeses following trauma. J Bone Joint Surg Am 1980;62(5):777–84.
20. O'Brien TS, Hart TS, Shereff MJ, et al. Open versus arthroscopic ankle arthrodesis: a comparative study. Foot Ankle Int 1999;20(6):368–74.
21. Stone JW. Arthroscopic ankle arthrodesis. Foot Ankle Clin 2006;11(2):361–8.
22. Collman DR, Kaas MH, Schuberth JM. Arthroscopic ankle arthrodesis: factors influencing union in 39 consecutive patients. Foot Ankle Int 2006;27:1079–85.
23. Winson IG, Robinson DE, Allen PE. Arthroscopic ankle arthrodesis. J Bone Joint Surg Br 2005;87(3):343–7.
24. Kats J, van Kampen A, de Waal-Malefijt MC. Improvement in technique for arthroscopic ankle fusion: results in 15 patients. Knee Surg Sports Traumatol Arthrosc 2003;11(1):46–9.
25. Dent CM, Patil M, Fairclough JA. Arthroscopic ankle arthrodesis. J Bone Joint Surg Br 1993;75(5):830–2.
26. Gougoulias NE, Agathangelidis FG, Parsons SW. Arthroscopic ankle arthrodesis. Foot Ankle Int 2007;28(6):695–706.
27. Ferkel RD, Hewitt M. Long-term results of arthroscopic ankle arthrodesis. Foot Ankle Int 2005;26(4):275–80.
28. Ogilvie-Harris DJ, Lieberman I, Fitsialos D. Arthroscopically assisted arthrodesis for osteoarthritic ankles. J Bone Joint Surg Am 1993;75(8):1167–74.
29. Zvijac JE, Lemak L, Schurhoff MR, et al. Analysis of arthroscopically assisted ankle arthrodesis. Arthroscopy 2002;18(1):70–5.
30. Schneider D. Arthroscopic ankle fusion. Arthroscopic Video J 1983;3.
31. Stetson WB, Ferkel RD. Ankle arthroscopy: II. Indications and results. J Am Acad Orthop Surg 1996;4(1):24–34.
32. Tang KL, Li QH, Chen GX, et al. Arthroscopically assisted ankle fusion in patients with end-stage tuberculosis. Arthroscopy 2007;23(9):919–22.

33. Myerson MS, Quill G. Ankle arthrodesis. A comparison of an arthroscopic and an open method of treatment. Clin Orthop Relat Res 1991;268:84–95.
34. Mann RA, Van Manen JW, Wapner K, et al. Ankle fusion. Clin Orthop Relat Res 1991;268:49–55.
35. Glick JM, Morgan CD, Myerson MS, et al. Ankle arthrodesis using an arthroscopic method: long-term follow-up of 34 cases. Arthroscopy 1996;12(4):428–34.
36. Jay RM. A new concept of ankle arthrodesis via arthroscopic technique. Clin Podiatr Med Surg 2000;17(1):147–57.
37. Monroe MT, Beals TC, Manoli A 2nd. Clinical outcome of arthrodesis of the ankle using rigid internal fixation with cancellous screws. Foot Ankle Int 1999;20(4): 227–31.
38. Crosby LA, Yee TC, Formanek TS, et al. Complications following arthroscopic ankle arthrodesis. Foot Ankle Int 1996;17:340–2.
39. Corso SJ, Zimmer TJ. Technique and clinical evaluation of arthroscopic ankle arthrodesis. Arthroscopy 1995;11:585–90.
40. Jerosch J, Steinbeck J, Schroder M, et al. Arthroscopically assisted arthrodesis of the ankle joint. Arch Orthop Trauma Surg 1996;115:182–9.
41. DeVriese L, Dereymaeker G, Fabry G. Arthroscopic ankle arthrodesis preliminary report. Acta Orthop Belg 1994;60:389–92.
42. Turan I, Wredmark T, Fellander-Tsai L. Arthroscopic ankle arthrodesis in rheumatoid arthritis. Clin Orthop 1995;320:110–4.
43. Blair HC. Comminuted fractures and fracture-dislocations of the body of the astragalus: operative treatment. Am J Surg 1943;59:37–43.
44. Brown CW, Orme TJ, Richardson HD. The rate of pseudoarthrosis (surgical nonunion) in patients who are smokers and patients who are nonsmokers; a comparison study. Spine 1986;11:942–3.
45. Glasman SD, Anagnost SC, Parker A, et al. The effect of cigarette smoking and smoking cessation on spinal fusion. Spine 2000;25:2608–15.
46. Haverstock BD, Mandracchia VJ. Cigarette smoking and bone healing: implication in foot and ankle surgery. J Foot Ankle Surg 1998;37:69–74.
47. Ishikawa SN, Murphy GA, Richardson EG. The effect of cigarette smoking on hindfoot fusions. Foot Ankle Int 2002;23:996–8.
48. Nolan J, Jenkins RA, Kurihara K, et al. The acute effects of cigareete smoke exposure on experimental skin flaps. Plast Reconstr Surg 1985;75:544–51.
49. Sherwin MA, Gastwirth CM. Detrimental effects of cigarette smoking on lower extremity wound healing. J Foot Surg 1990;29:84–7.
50. Cobb TK, Gabrielsen TA, Campbell DC 2nd, et al. Cigarette smoking and nonunion after ankle arthrodesis. Foot Ankle 1994;15:64–7.

Tibiotalocalcaneal Arthrodesis for Salvage of Severe Ankle Degeneration

Chul Kim, DPM, Alan R. Catanzariti, DPM, FACFAS*,
Robert W. Mendicino, DPM, FACFAS°

KEYWORDS

• Tibiotalocalcaneal • Arthrodesis • Ankle • Arthritis • Severe

Tibiotalocalcaneal (TTC) arthrodesis is a surgical option for patients who have severe ankle and hind foot arthrosis or malalignment (**Fig. 1**). Surgical techniques vary, and several forms of fixation have been developed, including intramedullary (IM) nails, screws, plates, and external fixators. Although the choice of fixation might be influenced by the surgeon's experience and expertise, certain variables dictate the ultimate choice. TTC arthrodesis is generally reserved for severe deformity at the ankle and subtalar joint (STJ) level, gross instability, Charcot reconstruction, insufficient talus not amenable to ankle fusion alone, or revisional surgery.[1–13] The procedure is reasonably predictable in select patients when traditional ankle fusion is not feasible or is inadequate to achieve correction. Studies have reported good outcomes clinically and radiographically for TTC arthrodesis with various types of fixation. This article provides a review of TTC arthrodesis, including preoperative evaluation, indications for the various procedures, operative techniques, ancillary procedures, and postoperative management.

PREOPERATIVE EVALUATION
History and Physical Examination

The patient's general health should be carefully assessed. Consultation with other medical disciplines is usually necessary before the procedure. Physical therapy should be ordered before surgery to evaluate the patient's ability to remain non-weight bearing for several months. Perioperative medical management of any comorbid conditions, such as diabetes mellitus, hypertension, or rheumatoid arthritis requiring chronic steroid therapy, should be implemented. Smoking cessation should be encouraged to increase the likelihood of primary union. Finally, as is the case with

Department of Foot and Ankle Surgery, The Western Pennsylvania Hospital, Pittsburgh, PA, USA
* Corresponding author. 1189 Lakemont Drive, Pittsburgh, PA 15243, USA.
E-mail address: acatanzariti@faiwp.com (A.R. Catanzariti).

Clin Podiatr Med Surg 26 (2009) 283–302
doi:10.1016/j.cpm.2008.12.009   podiatric.theclinics.com
0891-8422/08/$ – see front matter © 2009 Elsevier Inc. All rights reserved.

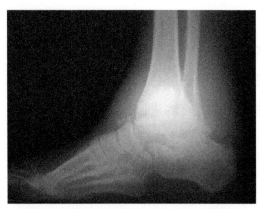

Fig. 1. Arthritic changes from previous trauma. The chronic nature of the arthritis causes extensive fibrotic changes of the joints and the bones.

any major reconstructive procedure, patients should have a thorough understanding of the magnitude of the operation and address any changes that need to be made at home and at work. A social work consultation is often helpful.

During the physical examination, one must assess the entire lower extremity. Preoperative considerations during the clinical examination include gross instability of the hind foot and ankle, deformity, degeneration of surrounding joints, and poor skin quality overlying the planned incision sites. Ankle range of motion is usually limited, with a sensation of crepitus or a palpable "click" (**Fig. 2**). Patients often complain of compensatory or postural pain in the STJ, lateral column pain, and cramping within the legs with long-standing arthrosis or deformity.

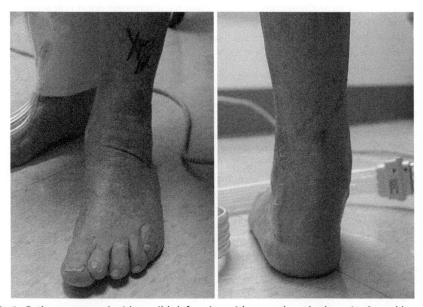

Fig. 2. Patient presented with a mild deformity, with warmth and edema in the ankle and hind foot. Radiographic changes of the ankle and the STJ correlate with the symptom complex.

Diagnostic Injections

Diagnostic injections can be useful for localizing the primary area of disease. The level of relief obtained with diagnostic injections can assist in preoperative planning and in procedure selection (**Fig. 3**). For example, with global pain secondary to combined subtalar and ankle joint disease, an ankle injection may provide only limited relief. After a subsequent injection into the STJ, however, the patient may experience complete resolution of pain. The examiner can conclude that the ankle joint and STJ are contributors to the overall level of pain and should both be addressed. Diagnostic injections allow the surgeon to determine the level of disease and serve as an effective nonoperative therapeutic intervention. Although the effect might be temporizing and variable from patient to patient, including a steroid, such as dexamethasone, can reduce inflammation and pain in the affected joints.

The exact technique and medications used during a diagnostic injection may vary. As long as an anesthetic agent and a water-soluble steroid are used, however, the desired result should be obtained. Injecting Xylocaine provides a quick onset for clinical diagnosis. Adding bupivacaine to the mixture provides an extended period of pain relief. The basic technique involves sterile preparation of the joint or joints to be injected. The surgeon then injects a local anesthetic and a water-soluble steroid into the ankle joint. After the injection, the patient begins range-of-motion exercises, followed by several minutes of ambulation. The amount of pain relief is then reassessed; if pain persists, other joints, such as the STJ, can be injected. This injection can also be performed under image intensification to improve accuracy.

ANCILLARY STUDIES AND PROCEDURES
Radiographic Evaluation

Patients with severe ankle degeneration may also have structural deformities. Using the realignment principles and the theory of 6° of freedom, preoperative limb deformity assessments should be performed. The level of deformity and the center of rotation of angulation (CORA) of the ankle and the STJ should be assessed to prevent proximal and distal articular degeneration.[14] Traditional radiographs and realignment views should be used. The long-leg calcaneal axial view and the hind foot alignment view assess the deformity and the degenerative process of the STJ and the ankle joint,

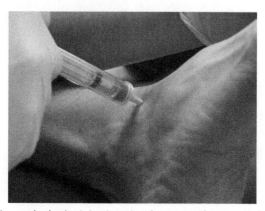

Fig. 3. Ankle injection and subtalar injection give short-term therapeutic benefit and assist in diagnosis.

respectively (**Fig. 4**).[15-17] The stress of surrounding joints can be reduced by accurately correcting the deformity.

Advanced Imaging

Preoperative advanced imaging is usually helpful to evaluate the deformity and the quality of the adjacent joints. Nonunion or malunion of previous surgery can be accurately diagnosed with the help of CT. The surgeon can also quantify the anticipated amount of osseous debridement and assess the structural quality of bone with the CT scan. MRI is beneficial in evaluating whether or not there is an avascular component to the degeneration. Additionally, as is the case with CT, MRI allows the surgeon to evaluate the amount of articular degeneration and assess the quality of the patient's subchondral bone. White blood cell (WBC)–labeled bone scans can be used to determine and rule out whether or not there is an infectious process occurring in the involved joints. This is especially important if there has been previous surgery or open wounds. WBC-labeled bone scans are highly specific for infection (**Fig. 5**). By using these imaging modalities, the surgeon can also exclude other types of arthropathies or diseases that adversely affect bone quality, such as Charcot neuroarthropathy or osseous neoplasm.

Biopsy

One should consider ruling out an infectious process or other forms of osseous pathologic conditions during revisional surgery. This is especially important when considering internal fixation or revising a nonunion. Biopsy should be considered in patients in whom infection is highly suspicious. Percutaneous biopsy performed under image intensification is a safe, effective, and technically simple preoperative procedure for

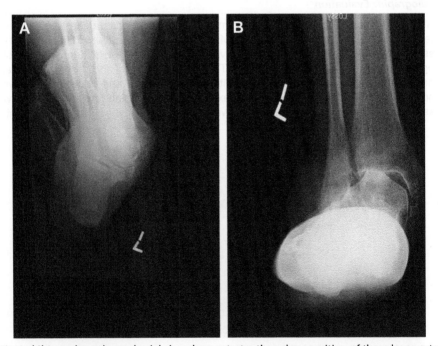

Fig. 4. (A) Long-leg calcaneal axial view demonstrates the valgus position of the calcaneus to the leg. (B) Hind foot alignment view demonstrates ankle valgus with instability.

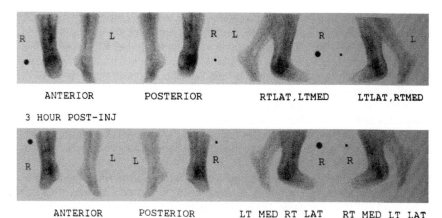

ANTERIOR   POSTERIOR   RTLAT,LTMED   LTLAT,RTMED

3 HOUR POST-INJ

ANTERIOR   POSTERIOR   LT MED RT LAT   RT MED LT LAT

Fig. 5. WBC-labeled bone scan shows osteomyelitis of the right hind foot and the ankle.

ruling out chronic infection or septic nonunion when radiographs are inconclusive (**Fig. 6**). Biopsy of the talus and tibia should be obtained from multiple areas to ensure a representative sample. Biopsy also allows the surgeon to rule out other diseases within the ankle joint, such as neuropathic arthropathies and rheumatoid arthritis. Biopsy is a dependable preoperative tool for ensuring that joint degeneration is the only process contributing to the patient's symptom complex.

Bone Grafting

Frequently, with severe degenerative changes of the ankle or in revisional operations, the surface area of the arthrodesis site is inadequate after correction of the deformity.

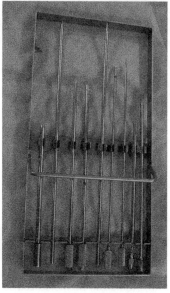

Fig. 6. Trephine biopsy instrument may help to diagnose the nature of the disease in the ankle and the STJ.

Angulations and length of bone for correction need to be in proper alignment, or the long-term prognosis of surgical intervention is poor. Furthermore, placement of internal hardware is often difficult when there is inadequate bone for internal fixation to purchase. Therefore, using bone grafts or orthobiologics is often necessary in TTC arthrodesis. Bone graft depends on the specific nature of the case. Iliac crest autograft is an ideal choice for providing structure and enhancing arthrodesis. Iliac crest grafts provide osteogenesis, osteoinduction, and osteoconduction, qualities that enhance arthrodesis. Therefore, autogenous iliac crest is ideal for revisional cases involving nonunion (**Fig. 7**A, B). Autografts can also be harvested from other areas, but iliac crest has a proved history with successful outcomes. Allograft bone can also be used to augment TTC arthrodesis (**Fig. 7**C, D).

Bone graft substitutes and orthobiologic materials, such as demineralized bone matrix, bone morphogenic proteins (BMPs), and platelet-rich plasma (PRP), may also be used in TTC arthrodesis. Surgeons should become familiar with their specific properties before implementing them in surgery. Although many products and options are available to augment the procedure, there is no substitute for the basic principles

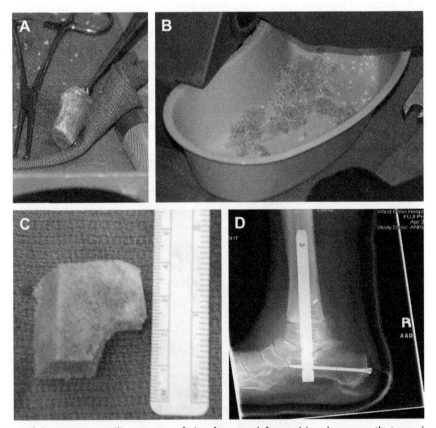

Fig. 7. (*A*) Autogenous iliac crest graft is often used for revisional surgery that requires osseous healing and support. (*B*) Fibula can be morselized to fill in defects and enhance arthrodesis. (*C, D*) Fresh femoral head allograft can be fashioned accordingly to provide structure in revisional surgery that requires restoration of height.

of arthrodesis recommended by Glissan:[18] adequate joint preparation, bone-to-bone apposition, appropriate position of the hind foot to the leg, and stable fixation.

SURGICAL OPTIONS FOR TIBIOTALOCALCANEAL ARTHRODESIS

There are several surgical techniques available for TTC arthrodesis. The choice of technique depends on many variables. The remainder of this article reviews the use of IM nail fixation, standard screw fixation, plate fixation, and external fixation for TTC arthrodesis.

INTRAMEDULLARY ROD FIXATION
Indications

TTC arthrodesis using IM nailing was described as early as 1906 by Lexer, who implanted a boiled corpse bone through the calcaneus, talus, and tibia.[19] Later, Albee[20] described using the fibula as a spike through the calcaneus and into the tibia. TTC arthrodesis with an IM nail should be reserved for patients who have significant deformity, gross instability, severe osteopenia, or revision (**Fig. 8**). Specific indications for an IM nail include patients who have failed ankle arthrodesis, arthroplasty, or total ankle replacement. Furthermore, patients who have skeletal defects after tumor resection, significant trauma, posttraumatic arthritis, avascular necrosis, rheumatoid arthritis, neuropathic arthropathy, or severe deformities secondary to clubfoot or neuromuscular disease are also candidates.[1–13]

Debridement of poor-quality bone to a level of healthy cancellous substrate is essential for arthrodesis, especially during revision. The IM nail provides a stable construct while bypassing the talus for fixation (**Fig. 9**). This eliminates the need to place screws from the tibia into the talus and is a reasonable option if the talus is

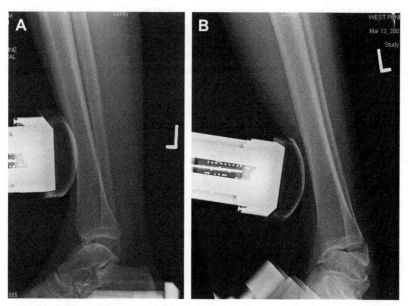

Fig. 8. Anteroposterior (*A*) and lateral (*B*) views of a patient with gross ankle and subtalar instability attributable to Ehrlos-Danlos syndrome, who has undergone previous ligamentous reconstruction for stabilization.

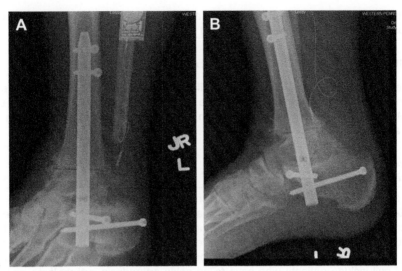

Fig. 9. (*A, B*) TTC arthrodesis with an IM nail.

unhealthy or requires extensive debridement. Other advantages of an IM nail include maintenance of length when sacrifice of the talus is necessary and stability in osteoporotic bone. TTC arthrodesis with an IM nail is a predictable surgical procedure when traditional forms of fixation have failed or are not practical.

Surgical Technique: Dissection and Joint Preparation

The authors prefer a lateral approach. The patient is usually placed in a supine position with appropriate bumps placed under the ipsilateral hip. The anterior surface of the patella should be perpendicular to the long axis of the tibia. An incision is made along the lateral ankle approximating the distal fibula and is curved at the tip of the lateral malleolus toward the sinus tarsi. The distal portion of the fibula is freed of all soft tissue attachments and is removed for appropriate exposure of the ankle joint and STJ. Care should be taken to protect the peroneal tendons, peroneal artery, and sural nerve. By evacuating the contents of the sinus tarsi and raising the extensor digitorum brevis muscle belly, exposure of the ankle and the STJ should be complete (**Fig. 10**A).

The joints should be resected appropriately through limited debridement or planning techniques (**Fig. 10**). The literature provides varying opinions regarding whether preparation of the STJ is even necessary.[21] The authors typically use limited debridement to prepare the STJ. Despite conflicting opinions in the literature, the authors have found that preparing the STJ seems to reduce the nonunion rate.

Planar resection is ideal to correct appropriately for deformity of the ankle joint. A second incision is usually necessary along the anterior aspect of the medial gutter of the ankle. This facilitates further debridement and visualization.

Realignment

The position of the TTC axis is observed and manipulated under image intensification. The calcaneus should be in a linear position with the tibia and the talus on the axial view. The position of the talus should be rectus and aligned with the tibia. The "center of the ankle joint," which is the middle portion of the talar dome on the anteroposterior view of the ankle and the lateral talar process on the lateral view, should align with the

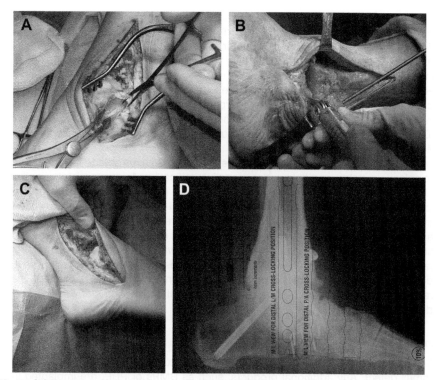

Fig. 10. (*A*) Exposure of the ankle and the STJ through the transfibular approach. (*B*) Preparation of the ankle joint with planar resection for the arthrodesis. (*C*) Prepared subtalar and ankle joint for arthrodesis. (*D*) Preoperative planning of the IM nail placement.

middiaphyseal line of the tibia. The bisection of the calcaneus should be parallel to the bisection of the distal one third of the tibia on the long-leg calcaneal axial view. The tibial bisection should also be 5 to 10 mm lateral to the calcaneus. Finding the CORA and performing an appropriate osteotomy or bone resection should be performed at the same time as the TTC arthrodesis when deformity of the distal tibia is present.[14–17] There should be a linear relation along the tibia, talus, and calcaneus, so that the foot is 90° to the leg, the foot is externally rotated slightly (10°–15°), and the heel is in rectus position to slight valgus. The correction of the deformity before delivering an IM nail is critical for success. Deviation may cause neurovascular damage to the pedal structures during the insertion. Additionally, malalignment may result in premature degeneration of the surrounding joints. If a structural bone graft is used, the graft and the joint surfaces should be fashioned accordingly, so that the deformity is corrected. An IM nail can only be used when collinear alignment of the tibia, talus, and calcaneus has been achieved.

Intramedullary Nail Placement

The IM nail is delivered after proper alignment. The interlocking screws are positioned differently according to the particular type of nail being used. An incision is placed on the central aspect of the plantar heel pad. Care is taken to avoid neurovascular and tendinous structures. Several articles report that the lateral plantar nerve is the most common structure damaged during IM nail delivery.[22–25] Flock and colleagues[23] recommended a mean distance of 2.1 cm proximal to the calcaneocuboid joint with careful protection of the nerve to the abductor digiti quinti. Stephenson and colleagues[24] proposed placing the incision at the intersection of two lines coinciding with anatomic landmarks. The first line is drawn from the second toe to the center of the heel, and the second line is placed at the junction of the anterior and middle thirds of the heel pad. According to these researchers, this approach did not produce any appreciable neurovascular damage. Roukis[25] later described translating the guide wire approximately 2.0 cm posterior to the "lower leg soft tissue outline" to allow proper positioning of the IM nail.

A guide wire and sequential reamers are introduced in a retrograde fashion through the calcaneus, talus, and tibia under image intensification. An appropriately sized nail is then delivered, and the distal interlocking screws are secured (**Fig. 11**). Compression through the joints is achieved, and the proximal interlocking screws are secured through an external alignment guide. This method prevents the distal aspect of the IM nail from protruding plantarly through the calcaneus as opposed to fixating the distal screws secondarily. Compression is avoided in revisional cases when larger bone grafts are used for structural support. Rotational stress of the arthrodesis sites should be checked; if rotational stress is present, supplemental fixation can be placed. There are reports in the literature discussing the use of staples or screws to achieve additional stiffness.[26–28]

Ancillary Procedures

The resected distal fibula can be used as a structural graft or morselized to pack a small defect. Any additional products, such as BMPs or PRP, are implanted into the arthrodesis. In cases of osteopenia or instability, a "neutralization" external fixator can be applied for additional stiffness. The external fixator provides excellent additional stability by preventing deforming forces, such torsion through the long axis of the tibia in the presence of osteopenia (**Fig. 12**).[29]

SCREW FIXATION

The preparation of the joints and alignment follow the same principles aforementioned in the previous sections. Screws can provide compression through the arthrodesis site, whereas an IM nail or plate may not because of its design. The authors use three or two screws through the STJ and ankle joint. A screw placed in an axial direction from the calcaneus to the tibia maintains alignment of the hind foot to the tibia. Additional screws are placed for stability and compression (**Fig. 13**). This design allows minimal osseous loss and is amenable to future revisional surgery if required.[26]

PLATE FIXATION

Plate fixation has been reported to achieve a good clinical and functional outcome for TTC arthrodesis. Depending on the design of the plate, the plates can be placed posterior, anterior, or lateral to the TTC arthrodesis site (**Fig. 14**). There is no distinct advantage or disadvantage among plates. Plates require more soft dissection relative to other forms of fixation. Extensive periosteal stripping may impede the vascular supply to the arthrodesis. Plate fixation provides stiffness to the construct, even more so than other types of fixation.[30–33]

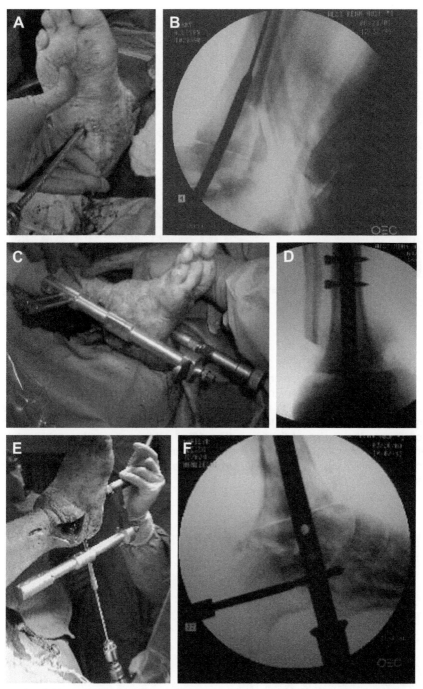

Fig. 11. (*A, B*) Placement of guide pin with proper alignment of the TTC relation and reaming for preparation of IM nail delivery. (*C, D*) Delivery of IM nail and the proximal interlocking screws through an external guide. (*E, F*) Placement of posterior-to-anterior interlocking screws.

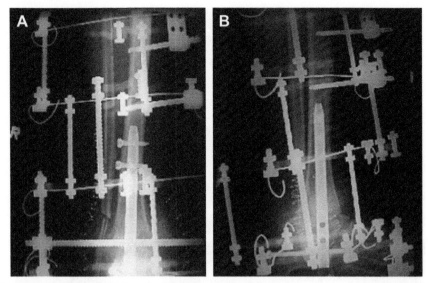

Fig. 12. (A, B) A neutralization frame over an IM nail provides additional stability through the arthrodesis site.

EXTERNAL FIXATION

External fixation, whether monolateral fixation or ring fixation, provides a stable construct with compression through the arthrodesis sites. Joint preparation and realignment are performed in a similar matter. With an external fixator, however, surgeons can provide stability to the construct by using small pins and compression according to the design of the frame (**Fig. 15**).[29] Additionally, with a proper stable frame construct, patients can ambulate with partial weight bearing. The negative aspects of using external fixation include pin site infection, difficult technique, and cost, for example.

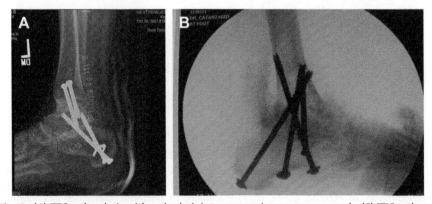

Fig. 13. (A) TTC arthrodesis with a single-joint compression screw approach. (B) TTC arthrodesis with a combined joint compression approach.

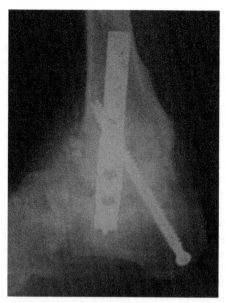

Fig. 14. TTC arthrodesis with a blade plate.

POSTOPERATIVE MANAGEMENT

A compressive dressing with splintage should be applied for 48 to 72 hours. A short-leg non–weight-bearing cast or other complete immobilizer should be applied until consolidation is seen on serial radiographs. If a dynamic compression IM nail was used, however, ambulation using a total contact cast can be initiated in 2 to 3 weeks. Elevation is important to limit edema and wound dehiscence. Gradual escalation of activity with physical therapy is encouraged after consolidation is complete. Loss of height to the postoperative limb may cause postural symptoms; thus, shoe modification or orthosis is often necessary. Lifts and rockers are applied to the affected limb for prevention of proximal and distal joint arthritis and postural symptoms.

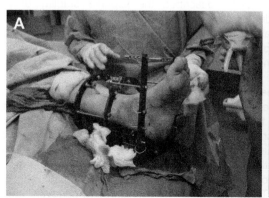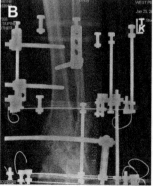

Fig. 15. (*A, B*) TTC arthrodesis using an external fixation device.

OUTCOMES
Osseous Consolidation

In 1994, Kile and colleagues[2] performed TTC arthrodesis with an IM nail on 30 patients. Many of them had been offered or considered amputations. Approximately 87% of the 30 patients reported satisfactory outcomes after the surgical procedure. Chou and colleagues[3] also reported on 48 fusions in 56 patients in a multicenter study. They found an average leg length discrepancy of 1.4 cm after surgery, which was treated with shoe modification and orthosis. In 2002, Millett and colleagues[34] achieved solid fusion in 14 of 15 patients who underwent TTC arthrodesis with an IM nail. The IM nail was used as a "salvage technique in complex posttraumatic or postsurgical settings" as opposed to other types of fixation because of its ability to bypass "insufficient bone stock." In 2005, Hammett and colleagues[35] reported on a series of 47 arthrodeses that demonstrated a healed arthrodesis site in a mean time of 4 months. In 2006, Goebel and colleagues[36] also achieved solid fusion in 25 (90%) of 29 patients. Seven of the patients had delayed union, however. Additionally, Pelton and colleagues[37] found an 88% fusion rate in 3.7 months. Mendicino and colleagues[38] found a 95% fusion rate in 4.1 months. In 2007, Niinimaki and colleagues[39] achieved radiographic and clinical fusion in 26 (76%) of 34 patients in a mean time of 16 weeks with a compressive retrograde IM nail. All investigators presented TTC arthrodesis with an IM nail as a successful form of fixation.

In 2006, Boer and colleagues[21] reported on 50 patients who had TTC with an IM nail without preparation of the STJ. All the ankles consolidated, whereas only two nonunions occurred in the STJ. These researchers questioned whether STJ preparation is necessary when the nonunion rate is so low.

Sekiya and colleagues[40] presented arthroscopy-assisted TTC arthrodesis in a patient who had rheumatoid arthritis in 2006. The ankle joint was prepared arthroscopically, whereas the STJ was prepared with percutaneous incision under fluoroscopic guidance. These researchers stated that patients who have rheumatoid arthritis have poor dermal conditions and that this approach may prevent wound dehiscence and infection.

Biomechanical Analysis and Alternative Fixation Techniques

The biomechanical parameters of the different fixation constructs are important. The design of the fixation, stiffness it provides by limiting micromotion, and compression, for example, are considered important factors for patients undergoing TTC arthrodesis.

In 2008, Muckley and colleagues[41] described the superior stability of the "compressed angle-stable locking" and "angle-stable locking" designs of the IM nail compared with the "statically locked" IM nail in cadaver and synthetic bone models. The first two designs provided more stability during cyclic testing, which includes a small range of motion in all three cardinal planes through the arthrodesis sites. Muckley and coworkers[42,43] also published a cadaveric study in which they tested these parameters plus the contact surface of compression of various IM nail designs. They found more stiffness and compression area in the compressed mode of the IM nail design as opposed to three-screw methods or a dynamic IM nail design.

Means and colleagues[44] described a posterior-to-anterior (PA) distal screw placement to provide a stiffer construct as opposed to transverse screw placement. The PA screws were inserted into the calcaneus and the talus. This cadaveric study showed higher fatigue endurance for the PA screw design as compared with the "traditional" transverse screws. This study was a reaffirmation of the cadaveric study by Mann and colleagues[45] in 2001, in which the PA calcaneal screw showed increased stiffness along the torque in the transverse plane. These investigators stated that the PA screw also provides similar results in osteopenic bone by purchasing more bone and higher quality bone in the sustentaculum tali area.

Different fixation techniques have been tested by many researchers regarding the stiffness of the construct for TTC arthrodesis. In 2005, Alfahd and colleagues[30] compared lateral blade plate fixation with an IM nail in a cadaveric study and showed a statistically significant reduction in internal rotation with the blade plate construct. Hanson and Cracchiolo[31] applied this principle in vivo, which showed 100% fusion in 10 patients in a mean time of 14.5 months. Later, Chodos and colleagues[32] biomechanically tested a blade plate versus a humeral locking plate in a cadaveric study and found that the locking plate provided higher initial stiffness, higher dorsiflexion and torsional load to failure, and lower construct deformation. This was tested as well in an in vivo model by Ahmad and colleagues,[33] who found 16 of 17 patients to have achieved fusion. In a synthetic bone study in 2005, Bennett and colleagues[26] found that a three-crossed cancellous screw technique provided the greatest stability with respect to micromotion as compared with IM nail and two-crossed cancellous screw groups. These researchers were able to achieve similar stability with an IM nail by adding a tibiotalar staple to the medial aspect of the ankle joint, however. This was contrary to the study by Fleming and colleagues,[46] who proposed that the IM nail with an interlocking screw provided more stability as compared with the three-cross cannulated screws in cadaveric models. Berend and colleagues[27] also proposed that the two-crossed lag screw fixation for TTC arthrodesis provided weaker resistance to bending and torsional forces compared with the IM nail construct.

COMPLICATIONS
Nonunion or Malunion

Nonunion or malunion is not uncommon, especially with revisional operations (**Fig. 16**).[47] Careful dissection to preserve vascular supplies to the osseous structures is important. Understanding anatomy when delivering the IM nail or minimizing dissection for plate placement can prevent vascular embarrassment. It is also important to prepare the joint surfaces adequately. One should visualize healthy bleeding cancellous surfaces for arthrodesis to take place. Appropriate use of the orthobiologic materials can augment the arthrodesis as well. Bone graft substitutes, BMPs, and other products are readily available. Revisional surgery with different fixation may be

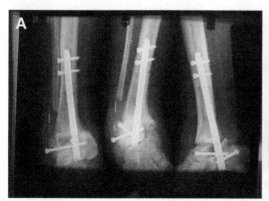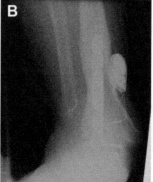

Fig. 16. (*A*) Nonunion of the TTC arthrodesis. (*B*) Malunion of the TTC arthrodesis with an IM nail. Note that the patient's calcaneus is still in valgus relation.

necessary if pseudoarthrosis occurs with an IM nail. Mudgal and Wilson[48] proposed using a blade plate in these situations, with additional debridement of the pseudoarthrosis. Proper alignment of the osseous structures, as previously discussed, can prevent degeneration of adjacent joints in the lower extremity. The TTC relation should be optimal for ambulation without significant stress compensation of the midtarsal joints or the proximal lower extremity joints.

Wound Dehiscence and Infection

Wound dehiscence and infection are possible complications especially with significant dissection with TTC arthrodesis. The areas of soft tissue tension, especially in

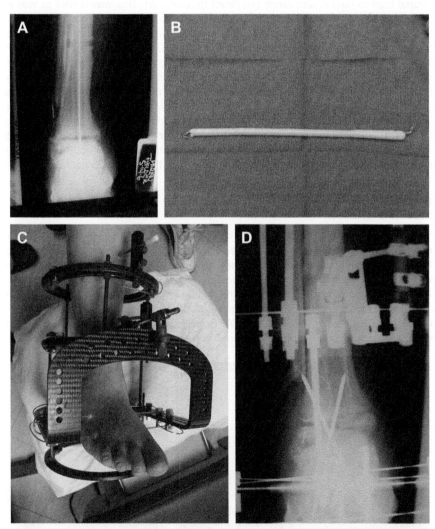

Fig. 17. (A, B) Placement of antibiotic-impregnated IM rod as a result of an infected previous IM rod and nonunion of the TTC arthrodesis. (C, D) Subsequent TTC arthrodesis with an external fixator device after resolution of the infection with long-term antibiosis and an antibiotic-impregnated rod.

severe deformity correction, should be understood. Tissue mobilization should be performed to allow proper healing of the surgical site. The IM nail can become infected, resulting in osteomyelitis. Bibbo and colleagues[49] suggested using an antibiotic-coated rod for salvage (**Fig. 17**). They were able to prevent amputation in four of five patients. Appropriate preoperative workup is important to prevent any intraoperative or postoperative complication regarding dehiscence and subsequent infection.

Stress Fracture

Stress fracture at the proximal interlocking screw in the tibia is a possible complication with IM nails (**Fig. 18**). Thordarson and Chang[50] reported 2 of 12 patients who developed stress risers in the proximal screw sites and were treated successfully with immobilization. They noted 7 patients who developed cortical hypertrophy in the areas, although no fracture occurred. Noonan and colleagues[51] found that long IM nails could prevent stress reaction in the tibial shaft. They found decreased strain on the posterior cortex of the tibia if the IM nail extended to the proximal tibial metaphysis. These investigators also suggested that there is a correlation between stress fracture and osteopenia.

Fat Embolism

Fat embolism syndrome is not a common complication from the IM nail in foot and ankle surgery. Fat embolism syndrome usually occurs in larger osseous structures, such as a femur IM nail. The possibility is always there, however, and early recognition of fat embolism syndrome is important in these patients.[52]

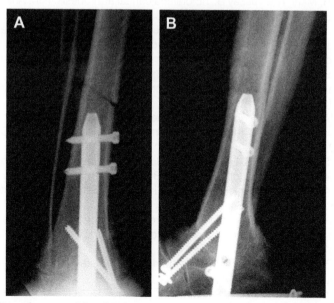

Fig. 18. (*A*) Stress fracture of the tibia in a patient status post-IM nail. (*B*) Fracture went on to heal uneventfully with immobilization.

Neurovascular Damage

Proper techniques should be used when inserting an IM nail. There are neurovascular structures at the insertion site in the middle of the calcaneal fat pad area. The most important factor is to position the hind foot to the tibia. Many anatomic and radiographic landmarks have been described to avoid the neurovascular structures.[22–25] Regardless of what technique the surgeon prefers, careful dissection through the soft tissue to visualize the calcaneus and placement of the IM nail is important. Vascular compromise can result in nonunion and wound dehiscence, whereas nerve injury can cause postoperative paresthesias that can be difficult to manage.

SUMMARY

TTC arthrodesis is a successful and proved surgical procedure for patients who have significant arthritic changes, deformity, and failed previous operations. Surgical technique varies depending on the type of fixation. Basic surgical principles should not be violated. Correction of the deformity with appropriate joint preparation and stable fixation is important for a good outcome. Other adjunctive materials, such as bone growth stimulators and orthobiologics, should be used appropriately to ensure adequate primary arthrodesis.

REFERENCES

1. Russotti GM, Johnson KA, Cass JR. Tibiotalocalcaneal arthrodesis for arthritis and deformity of the hind part of the foot. J Bone Joint Surg Am 1988;70(9): 1304–7.
2. Kile TA, Donnelly RE, Gehrke JC, et al. Tibiotalocalcaneal arthrodesis with an intramedullary device. Foot Ankle Int 1994;15:669–73.
3. Chou LB, Mann RA, Yaszay B. Tibiotalocalcaneal arthrodesis. Foot Ankle Int 2000; 21(10):804–8.
4. Fox IM, Shapero C, Kennedy A. Tibiotalocalcaneal arthrodesis with intramedullary interlocking nail fixation. Clin Podiatr Med Surg 2000;17(1):19–31.
5. Hopgood P, Kumar R, Wood PLR, et al. Ankle arthrodesis for failed total ankle replacement. J Bone Joint Surg Br 2006;88-B(8):1032–8.
6. Kitaoka HB, Romness DW. Arthrodesis for failed ankle arthroplasty. J Arthroplasty 1992;7(3):277–84.
7. Papa JA, Myerson MS. Pantalar and tibiotalocalcaneal arthrodesis for post-traumatic osteoarthrosis of the ankle and hindfoot. J Bone Joint Surg 1992;74-A(7): 1042–9.
8. Levine SE, Myerson MS, Lucas P, et al. Salvage of pseudoarthrosis after tibiotalar arthrodesis. Foot Ankle Int 1997;18(9):580–5.
9. Felix NA, Kitaoka HB. Ankle arthrodesis in patients with rheumatoid arthritis. Clin Orthop Relat Res 1998;349:58–64.
10. Acosta R, Ushiba J, Cracchiolo A. The results of a primary and staged pantalar arthrodesis and tibiotalocalcaneal arthrodesis in adult patients. Foot Ankle Int 2000;21(3):182–94.
11. Kelly IP, Nunley JA. Treatment of stage 4 adult acquired flatfoot. Foot Ankle Clin 2001;6(1):167–78.
12. De Smet K, De Brauwer V, Burssens P, et al. Tibiocalcaneal Marchetti-Vicenzi nailing in revision arthrodesis for posttraumatic pseudoarthrosis of the ankle. Acta Orthop Belg 2003;69(1):42–8.

13. Muir D, Angliss RD, Nattrass GR, et al. Tibiotalocalcaneal arthrodesis for severe calcaneovalgus deformity in cerebral palsy. J Pediatr Orthop 2005;25(5):651–6.
14. Paley D, Herzenberg JE. Principles of deformity correction. New York: Springer-Verlag; 2002.
15. Mendicino RW, Catanzariti AR, Reeves CL, et al. A systematic approach to evaluation of the rearfoot, ankle, and leg in reconstructive surgery. J Am Podiatr Med Assoc 2005;95(1):2–12.
16. Mendicino RW, Lamm BM, Catanzariti AR, et al. Realignment arthrodesis of the rearfoot and ankle. J Am Podiatr Med Assoc 2005;95(1):60–71.
17. Lamm BM, Mendicino RW, Catanzariti AR, et al. Static rearfoot alignment a comparison of clinical and radiographic measures. J Am Podiatr Med Assoc 2005;95(1):26–33.
18. Glissan DJ. The indications for inducing fusion at the ankle joint by operation with description of two successful techniques. Aust N Z J Surg 1949;19:64–71.
19. Adams JC. Arthrodesis of the ankle joint: experiences with the transfibular approach. J Bone Joint Surg Br 1948;39:506–11.
20. Albee FH. Bone-graft surgery. Philadelphia: WB Saunders; 1915. p. 335.
21. Boer R, Mader K, Pennig D, et al. Tibiotalocalcaneal arthrodesis using a reamed retrograde locking nail. Clin Orthop Relat Res 2007;463:151–6.
22. McGarvey WC, Trevino SG, Baxter DE, et al. Tibiotalocalcaneal arthrodesis: anatomic and technical considerations. Foot Ankle Int 1998;19(6):363–9.
23. Flock TJ, Ishikawa S, Hecht PJ, et al. Heel anatomy for retrograde tibiotalocalcaneal roddings: a roentgenographic and anatomic analysis. Foot Ankle Int 1997;18(4):233–5.
24. Stephenson KA, Kile TA, Graves SC. Estimating the insertion site during retrograde intramedullary tibiotalocalcaneal arthrodesis. Foot Ankle Int 1996;17(12):781–2.
25. Roukis TS. Determining the insertion site for retrograde intramedullary nail fixation of tibiotalocalcaneal arthrodesis: a radiographic and intraoperative anatomical landmark analysis. J Foot Ankle Surg 2006;45(4):227–34.
26. Bennett GL, Cameron B, Njus G, et al. Tibiotalocalcaneal arthrodesis: a biomechanical assessment of stability. Foot Ankle Int 2005;26(7):530–6.
27. Berend ME, Glisson RR, Nunley JA. A biomechanical comparison of intramedullary nail and crossed lag screw fixation for tibiotalocalcaneal arthrodesis. Foot Ankle Int 1997;18(10):639–43.
28. Chiodo CP, Acevedo JI, Sammarco VJ, et al. Intramedullary rod fixation compared with blade-plate-and-screw fixation for tibiotalocalcaneal arthrodesis: a biomechanical investigation. J Bone Joint Surg 2003;85-A(12):2425–8.
29. Kalish S, Fleming J, Weinstein R. External fixators for elective rearfoot and ankle arthrodesis techniques and indications. Clin Podiatr Med Surg 2003;20:65–96.
30. Alfahd U, Roth SE, Stephen D, et al. Biomechanical comparison of intramedullary nail and blade plate fixation for tibiotalocalcaneal arthrodesis. J Orthop Trauma 2005;19(10):703–8.
31. Hanson TW, Cracchiolo A. The use of a 95 blade plate and a posterior approach to achieve tibiotalocalcaneal arthrodesis. Foot Ankle Int 2002;23(8):704–10.
32. Chodos MD, Parks BG, Schon LC, et al. Blade plate compared with locking plate for tibiotalocalcaneal arthrodesis: a cadaver study. Foot Ankle Int 2008;29(2):219–24.
33. Ahmad J, Pour AE, Raikin SM. The modified use of a proximal humeral locking plate for tibiotalocalcaneal arthrodesis. Foot Ankle Int 2007;28(9):977–83.

34. Millett PJ, O'Malley MJ, Tolo ET, et al. Tibiotalocalcaneal fusion with a retrograde intramedullary nail: clinical and functional outcomes. Am J Orthop 2002;31(9): 531–6.

35. Hammett R, Hepple S, Forster B, et al. Tibiotalocalcaneal (hindfoot) arthrodesis by retrograde intramedullary nailing using a curved locking nail: the results of 52 procedures. Foot Ankle Int 2005;26(10):810–5.

36. Goebel M, Gerdesmeyer L, Muckley T, et al. Retrograde intramedullary nailing in tibiotalocalcaneal arthrodesis: a short-term prospective study. J Foot Ankle Surg 2005;45(2):98–106.

37. Pelton K, Hofer JK, Thordarson DB. Tibiotalocalcaneal arthrodesis using a dynamically locked retrograde intramedullary nail. Foot Ankle Int 2007;27(10):759–63.

38. Mendicino RW, Catanzariti AR, Saltrick KR, et al. Tibiotalocalcaneal arthrodesis with retrograde intramedullary nailing. J Foot Ankle Surg 2004;43(2):82–6.

39. Niinimaki TT, Klemola TM, Leppilahti JI. Tibiotalocalcaneal arthrodesis with a compressive retrograde intramedullary nail: a report of 34 consecutive patients. Foot Ankle Int 2007;28(4):431–4.

40. Sekiya H, Horii T, Kariya Y, et al. Arthroscopic-assisted tibiotalocalcaneal arthrodesis using an intramedullary nail with fins: a case report. J Foot Ankle Surg 2006; 45(4):266–70.

41. Muckley T, Hoffmeier K, Klos K, et al. Angle-stable and compressed angle-stable locking for tibiotalocalcaneal arthrodesis with retrograde intramedullary nails. J Bone Joint Surg Am 2008;90-A(3):620–7.

42. Muckley T, Ullm S, Petrovitch A, et al. Comparison of two intramedullary nails for tibiotalocalcaneal fusion: anatomic and radiographic considerations. Foot Ankle Int 2007;28(5):605–13.

43. Muckley T, Eichorn S, Hoffmeier K, et al. Biomechanical evaluation of primary stiffness of tibiotalocalcaneal fusion with intramedullary nails. Foot Ankle Int 2007; 28(2):224–31.

44. Means KR, Parks BG, Nguyen A, et al. Intramedullary nail fixation with posterior-to-anterior compared to transverse distal screw placement for tibiotalocalcaneal arthrodesis: a biomechanical investigation. Foot Ankle Int 2006;27(12):1137–42.

45. Mann MR, Parks BG, Pak SS, et al. Tibiotalocalcaneal arthrodesis: a biomechanical analysis of the rotational stability of the Biomet ankle arthrodesis. Foot Ankle Int 2001;22(9):731–3.

46. Fleming SS, Moore TJ, Hutton WC. Biomechanical analysis of hindfoot fixation using an intramedullary rod. J South Orthop Assoc 1998;7(1):19–26.

47. Cooper PS. Complications of ankle and tibiotalocalcaneal arthrodesis. Clin Orthop Relat Res 2001;391:33–44.

48. Mudgal CS, Wilson MG. Revision tibiotalocalcaneal arthrodesis after a failed intramedullary rod: a technique tip. Foot Ankle Int 1999;20(3):210–1.

49. Bibbo C, Lee S, Anderson RB, et al. Limb salvage: the infected retrograde tibiotalocalcaneal intramedullary nail. Foot Ankle Int 2003;24(5):420–5.

50. Thordarson DB, Chang D. Stress fractures and tibial cortical hypertrophy after tibiotalocalcaneal arthrodesis with an intramedullary nail. Foot Ankle Int 1999; 20(8):497–500.

51. Noonan T, Pinzur M, Paxinos O, et al. Tibiotalocalcaneal arthrodesis with a retrograde intramedullary nail: a biomechanical analysis of the effect of nail length. Foot Ankle Int 2005;26(4):304–8.

52. Talbot M, Schemitsch EH. Fat embolism syndrome: history, definition, epidemiology. Injury 2006;37(Suppl 4):S3–7.

Total Ankle Arthroplasty: Indications and Avoiding Complications

Jerome K. Steck, DPM, FACFAS[a,b,*], Jason B. Anderson, DPM[b]

KEYWORDS

- Arthroplasty • Ankle • Arthritis • Ankle degenerative disease
- Total ankle arthroplasty (TAA) • Total ankle replacement (TAR)

Total ankle arthroplasty (TAA) is an exciting frontier in the management of end-stage ankle arthrosis. Although ankle arthrodesis is still considered the gold standard in the treatment of end-stage ankle arthritis, this standard is being challenged, as many short-term as well as long-term problems are associated with ankle arthrodesis,[1–8] and advancements in TAA continue to improve. A viable and reliable arthroplasty is an invaluable alternative to the patient suffering from end-stage ankle osteoarthritis. TAA has a steep learning curve; surgeons and manufacturers continue to develop and improve implants and instrumentation to dampen this curve. Not unlike any other difficult endeavor, many hours of study and training are needed to develop clinical acumen and surgical fortitude in the arena of TAA. In this regard, McGill University neurologist Dr. Daniel Levitin has expressed the following:

> "Ten thousand hours of practice is required to achieve the level of mastery associated with being a world-class expert — in anything. In study after study, of composers, basketball players, fiction writers, ice skaters, concert pianists, chess players, master criminals, and what have you, this number comes up again and again. Ten thousand hours is the equivalent to roughly three hours per day, or twenty hours per week, of practice over ten years. It seems that it takes the brain this long to assimilate all that it needs to know to achieve true mastery."

Currently, three main designs of TAA are approved by the FDA: the Agility (DePuy), Salto Talaris (Tournier) and Inbone (Wright). Although I am familiar with each, I have the most experience with the Agility, including 9 years and over 400 cases. In addition, I spent three years with the inventor of the Agility, Dr. Frank Alvine, a true master of TAA. Thus, in this article I refer primarily to the Agility; however, the underlying

[a] Southern Arizona Orthopaedics, University of Arizona, Tucson, AZ 85710, USA
[b] Jewish Hospital, University of Louisville, 6567 East Carondelet Drive, Suite 415, Tuscon, AZ 85710, USA
* Corresponding author.
E-mail address: jksteck@hotmail.com (J.K. Steck).

Clin Podiatr Med Surg 26 (2009) 303–324
doi:10.1016/j.cpm.2009.02.001
0891-8422/09/$ – see front matter © 2009 Elsevier Inc. All rights reserved.

podiatric.theclinics.com

principles surrounding each system are similar and I will focus on generalities rather than individual nuances.

HISTORY

A detailed review of the history of ankle replacements is not documented here, but the evolution is quite remarkable and fascinating.[8] Early cemented TAA designs bred complications and revisions. Respect for the kinematics and the biomechanical demand of the ankle was underestimated.

First-generation implant designs relied on a cemented, constrained configuration that transmitted a great deal of force across the bone–cement interface. Revision rates were as high as 41% in some studies.[9–11] Takakura and colleagues[12] reported component loosening in 85% of cemented ankles by 5 years.

Short and midterm results of the second-generation (implants, which are usually cementless, semiconstrained in the United States and mobile-bearing in Europe, improve results with respect to revision rates.[13] In a review of 306 TAAs, Spirt[14] reported a reoperation rate of 28%, with heterotopic bone debridement being the most common revisional procedure, whereas 10% required component replacement. It is important to note that the study reinforced the idea that young age (≤54) had a negative effect on reoperation rates and failure. Contrary to an earlier study that found no significant differences between age groups.[15,16]

Pyevich[13] reported a 6% revision rate with second-generation TAA, and a recent meta-analysis of second generation implants reported a 7% revision rate, less than arthrodesis.[17]

Due in part to lack of long-term follow-up studies, early TAA designs failed to live up to the expectations and standards in total joint arthroplasty in the orthopedic community.[12,17,18] A recurring theme among first-generation implants was subsidence of the tibial component into the relatively weak lateral distal bone. The Agility design has addressed this issue by spanning the cortical bone of the lateral tibia and medial fibula with the integration of a syndesmotic fusion.

New designs and a better understanding of kinematics, patient selection, and implant methods have lead to a rejuvenated interest in TAA.[4,19,20] Although improved design has decreased the frequency of revision, the causes and inherent difficulty associated with revision TAA remain the same. Poor soft tissue coverage, potential loss of bone stock, and limited "off the shelf" revision components make revision challenging; however, the majority of complications in TAA can now be revised, making conversion to a fusion or amputation rare in experienced hands.

INDICATIONS AND CONTRAINDICATIONS
Patient Selection

The initial step in any arthroplasty is patient selection; this process is paramount to a successful outcome. Each patient encounter is unique. A thorough history and physical examination must be performed and conservative treatment exhausted. The surgeon must gather all available information and remain astute in determining whether a patient is a viable candidate. The indications and contraindications listed in **Box 1** are merely guidelines; extreme attention to detail and individualization is absolutely necessary. Extended training or a fellowship would serve to increase clinical acumen and surgical skills associated with perioperative management of TAA.

In performing an overall patient assessment, all risk factors must be accounted for. As with any elective surgery, if the risks outweigh the benefits, an alternative treatment is selected, and should be considered if several relative contraindications exist. However,

Box 1
Indications, relative contraindications, and absolute contraindications for TAA

Indications

1. Age > 55

2. Low physical demand

3. Good bone stock

4. Neurovascular status intact

5. No immunosuppression

6. Ankle alignment neutral or able to be reduced to neutral intraoperatively

7. Competent deltoid

8. Arthritic degeneration secondary to

    a. Inflammatory arthritis

    b. Osteoarthritis

    c. Traumatic arthritis

    d. Septic arthritis (if > 1 year since infection; CRP, ESR normal; and biopsy and aspiration negative for acute or chronic infection)

Relative contraindications

1. Avascular necrosis of talus if necrotic portion of talus will be excised with bony cuts

2. Age < 55

3. Poor bone stock

4. Immunosuppression

5. Smoking

6. Ankle deformity (varus, valgus, procurvatum, recurvatum)

7. History of septic ankle

8. History of severe trauma with bone loss

9. Diabetes

10. Obesity

11. Workman compensation cases

12. Osteoporosis

Absolute contraindications

1. High physical demands (eg, construction worker; running, jumping)

2. Poor distal vascular supply

3. Significant neuropathy from any cause

4. Incompetent deltoid or nonreconstructable deformity

5. Suspicion of infection

6. Severe soft tissue compromise (ie, multiple previous incisions, flaps)

7. Neuromuscular deficit/paralysis

8. Noncompliance

9. Avascular necrosis of entire talar body

patients who have several relative contraindications may be poor surgical candidates regardless of the selected treatment. For example, a meta-analysis by Haddad and colleagues[17] demonstrated that the complication, revision, and below–the-knee amputation (BKA) rates were higher in ankle fusion than in TAA. In general, however, complications associated with TAA have a higher morbidity than those seen with ankle fusion.[7]

Several authors consider TAA to be contraindicated in patients with diabetes mellitus (DM). Many of these concerns are justified in light of the tenuous blood supply surrounding the ankle. The effects of DM on macro- and microcirculation and neuropathy in the foot and ankle are significantly more profound than in the hip or knee. Thus, TAA in DM patients presents a far greater risk than does total hip or knee arthroplasty.

I do not believe that DM in and of itself is an absolute contraindication to TAA. Characteristically, patients who have DM possess relative risk factors that preclude them from TAA (**Box 1**) The progression of these factors consists of compromised blood supply, poor tissue perfusion, and advancing neuropathy. In some circumstances, DM patients without neuropathy may be reasonable candidates for TAA. However, significant neuropathy, diabetic or otherwise, is an absolute contraindication to TAA. Increased complications will arise when performing TAA on patients who have DM and I do not advocate the beginning TAA surgeon attempt it.

Preoperative Considerations

A thorough preoperative physical examination is critical. In addition to the overall medical stability of the patient, the surgeon should check for remote signs of infection. This includes, but is not limited to, dentition, any open lesion of the extremities, previous scars, urinary tract infections, and upper respiratory infections. If any of these are present the case should be cancelled until the issue is resolved.

An extensive informed consent should include a thorough review of all of the risks, benefits, possible complications, expected outcomes, and treatment alternatives. A discussion of what will take place if infection or other complications occur is vitally important and should include the possibilities of additional surgery, external fixation, extended convalescence, chronic pain, complex regional pain syndrome (CRPS), revision, intraoperative conversion to fusion, and amputation.

Radiographic Evaluation

Review of preoperative radiographs should include evaluation of overall bone stock; if significant osteopenia is suspected, bone densitometry should be considered.

Skeletal deformity that can affect the function of a TAA can occur above, at, or below the level of the ankle. This deformity needs to be identified and if possible corrected either before or during joint implantation as residual deformity will negatively affect the function of the implant. Some deformities are too severe to correct and arthrodesis should be performed (**Fig. 1**). Multiple simultaneous adjunctive procedures should be approached with caution. For example, a triple arthrodesis for a pes planus deformity and a TAA can be done, but due to increased surgical time and proximity of incisions, wound dehiscence is more likely.

Cystic changes are common with end stage arthrosis of the ankle and are often more extensive than they appear on plain radiographs. If cysts are suspected, a CT scan is indicated. Large cysts can alter surgical planning dramatically. The patient in **Fig. 2** required a custom stemmed talar component to bypass this large cyst; interestingly, this cyst appeared small and inconsequential on standard radiographs.

Previous hardware, especially in the medial malleolous, may need to be removed before TAA, as the resultant bone void may act as a stress riser.

Adjacent joints should be evaluated for deformity and arthrosis (**Fig. 3**).

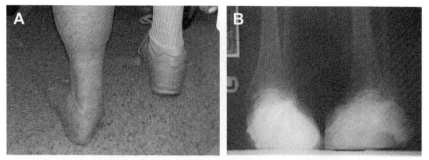

Fig.1. (*A*) Clinical photograph of a prospective TAA patient. (*B*) Preoperative AP and mortise radiograph. The amount of valgus as well as the ball-and-socket ankle joint should raise significant concerns regarding this patient's candidacy for TAA, and arthrodesis should be performed.

SURGICAL CONSIDERATIONS

Surgeon experience and proper patient selection are consistently the most important factors in determining favorable outcomes. Schuberth and Myerson have independently reported that outcomes significantly improve with surgeon experience.[10,11,21–25] Haskell and Mann[21] also demonstrated a decrease in perioperative complications with increasing surgeon experience. It is my belief that a so-called "learning curve" is a polite way of reporting considerable complications. Surgeons possess the power to significantly help or hurt people and it is our responsibility to acquire adequate training so as to minimize complications. It is the responsibility of the manufacturers, in collaboration with experienced surgeons, to continue to improve instrumentation and techniques that enable reproducible results, and thus minimize morbidity to the patient. Comprehensive surgeon training, including observation of, and proctoring by, an experienced surgeon are necessary for adequate TAA training.[26] Saltzman and colleagues[22] suggested that none of the current modalities for training TAA surgeons are statistically different in predicting patient outcomes. These investigators emphasize, however, that initial use of TAA be approached with caution and

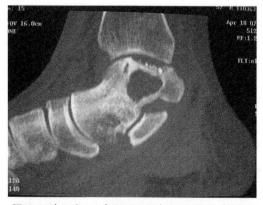

Fig. 2. Preoperative CT scan showing a large cyst that appeared quite small on plain film radiographs. This patients procedure was changed due to this CT and had a custom stemmed talar component made to bypass this large cyst.

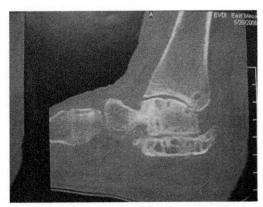

Fig. 3. In addition to an ankle replacement, the subtalar joint needs to be addressed in this patient who has end-stage osteoarthritis of both joints.

serious consideration. It is the responsibility of the surgeon to identify and understand their surgical limitations as well as the limitations of the implant.

Development of a surgical team is invaluable. This team should include: assistants (ideally, two), an experienced scrub technician, a circulating nurse product representative, and a radiology technician. The ability to work repeatedly with these individuals will significantly decrease OR time as well as decrease surgeon frustration. For example, teaching the system to the scrub tech during the case is fraught with difficulty. Many manufacturers will provide a saw bone or cadaveric lab experience for the team in anticipation of their first case; this should be requested before the surgeon's first case and repeated as needed for new staff. In general, the shorter the tourniquet and operating time, the lower the complication rate.

TAA is both an ankle surgery and a total joint surgery. Techniques and principles from both disciplines must be melded together. Concentrating only on foot and ankle surgery may lead to oversight of important principles relating to total joint surgery and the risk of a devastating infection is increased. Conversely, the total joint surgeon may neglect a foot or leg deformity that can lead to imbalance of the prosthesis and result in catastrophic failure. The properly trained TAA surgeon must be well-versed in each discipline for optimal outcomes.

Surgical Technique

The steep learning curve is due primarily to the demanding and intricate nature of the procedure. I have likened learning the surgical technique for TAA to learning gross anatomy: none of the concepts are difficult to learn by themselves, just as learning one bone or muscle in anatomy is not difficult, but putting them all together in a short amount of time, often under duress, is much more challenging. Although the details of surgical technique are not the main focus of this article, this section discusses surgical principles pertinent to all TAA designs. (Each implant available has a unique technique guide and is not covered individually here.)

Major perioperative elements
The major steps are shown pictorially in (**Fig. 4**A–I).

Skin preparation Skin preparation can be achieved with a standard betadine preparation or with products such as ChloraPrep (Cardinalhealth), which has been shown to have added benefits of extended antimicrobial action versus standard preparation.[18,27] Regardless of the choice in skin preparation, care must be taken to thoroughly complete this step. I often perform this step myself after repeatedly witnessing poor skin preparation, especially in the interdigital spaces. Coverage of all exposed skin with an adhesive skin covering is recommended, with the exception of patients with fragile skin (eg, rheumatoid arthritis), because removal of the adhesive drape can cause skin damage. The forefoot, including the toes, should never be exposed. If accessory procedures are required, the anterior ankle incision is closed before proceeding to the next procedure.

Skin and soft tissue handling The anterior incision is fragile, and dehiscence at the level of the ankle joint is the most common when dehiscense occurs. Incisions should be of adequate length to prevent excessive retraction. Even with appropriate skin incisions, the retraction is still extensive (**Fig. 4**D, G and I). Full thickness flaps should be created and undermining avoided. Dissection is advanced between the interval of the tibialis anterior and the extensor halluxis longus. The anterior tibial vessels and deep peroneal nerve should be retracted laterally (**Fig. 4**C).

Bone cuts Placement of an alignment guide and cutting jig is the "point of no return" and should be done with attention to all prescribed detail (**Fig. 4**E). Once the bone cuts are made, it is very difficult, if not impossible, to make corrections. Large saw blades are used with large excursions and one must protect the malleoli. The posterior tibial tendon is taut against the posterior tibia, and plunging of the saw blade will easily cut this tendon. The posterior medial neurovascular structures are also in danger due to proximity to the bone cuts (**Fig. 4**G).

Ligament tension Ligament tension across the joint is mandatory and obtained through a variety of techniques. In the Agility ankle tension is obtained through an external fixator and the joint is distracted to the deltoid endpoint and then backed off two millimeters to allow for porous coated implants, meaning that the deltoid is now properly tensioned and the bone cuts can now be made (**Fig. 4**D). In the Salto Talaris, and Inbone, increasing thicknesses of poly can be inserted to tension the joint. Regardless of the technique, failure to do this leaves a lax joint doomed to failure.

Bone quality and use of cement Patients who are elderly or who have rheumatoid arthritis or diabetes often present with poor bone quality. Although TAA implants are designed to encourage bony ingrowth, they are only FDA-approved for cemented application. Using cement is difficult for TAA and most surgeons will not cement the prosthesis. However, in patients with severe osteoporosis, cement is advisable to create a stable implant. Caution must be used when using cement, because more bone needs to be resected to make room for the cement itself and any excessive cement posteriorly is very difficult, if not impossible, to retrieve causing irritation to the tendonous or neurovascular structures.

Closure Closure is done according to surgeon preference with special care taken to avoid excessive tension on the skin. I find it best to use a simple or running suture in the skin rather than staples. A drain is controversial; I prefer not to use a drain as arthrosis is not very uncommon.

Postoperative Treatment

Postoperative convalescence can be a challenge. Most TAA devices rely on bony ingrowth to occur at the prosthesis–bone interface; requiring the patient to remain nonweight-bearing for at least 6 weeks, this can be difficult for the elderly and frail

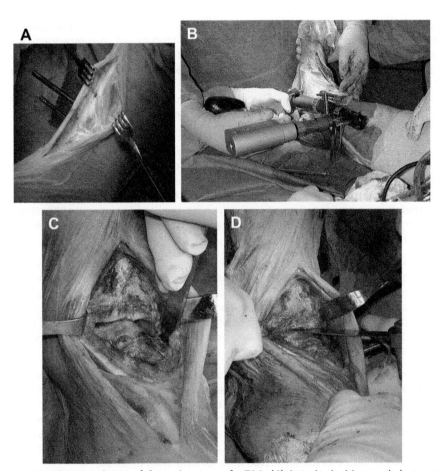

Fig. 4. Step-by-step photos of the major steps of a TAA. (*A*) Anterior incision made between the anterior tibial and extensor hallucis longus tendons. Note the superficial peroneal nerve in the wound and the amount of retraction. (*B*) Application of monolateral external fixator used to tension the joint and for stabilization. (*C*) Full exposure of the anterior ankle. This patient has a varus deformity. (*D*) Finding the deltoid endpoint. This step ensures that the ligaments surrounding the ankle will be out to length and will support the TAA. It is achieved in the Agility system shown here by distracting the external fixator. (*E*) Application of the alignment guide and cutting jig. This step is the point of no return and attention to detail is paramount. (*F*) Typical amount of bone resected. To the left is the tibia and to the right is the talus. In this patient, the total amount of resected bone measured 1.4 cm. (*G*) After the bone cuts have been made (medial is to the right). Also note the posterior tibial tendon posteriomedial and the slot in the medial distal tibia for the tibial component. (*H*) Trial placement. These components should fit loosely due to lack of porous coating. (*I*) Final implant placement. These fit snugly due to the porous coating on the final implant.

patient. If there is any question about their ability to be independent, or if they live alone, convalescence in a rehabilitation or skilled nursing facility should be seriously considered, even if the patient has a healthy support system. In my experience, patients who choose a rehabilitation or skilled nursing facility healed faster, had fewer

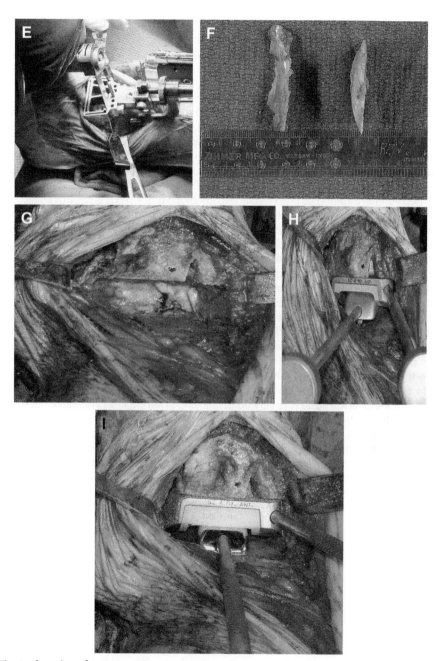

Fig. 4. (*continued*)

complications, and better overall outcomes than those who recovered at home and struggled to be non-weight bearing.

Strict adherence to preoperative and operative protocols and techniques can all be for naught if attention for detail is lost during the postoperative course. Obviously there are variations in postoperative protocol from surgeon to surgeon. The key, however, is close and frequent follow-up and appropriate monitoring of the wound.

A dichotomy arises postoperatively between wound healing and early ankle range of motion (ROM). Extrapolating from hip and knee arthroplasty philosophy, earlier ROM equals increased overall ROM; however, in TAA, the anterior wound is fragile and ROM should not occur at the expense of wound healing. For this reason, I immobilize the ankle in a posterior splint for 2 weeks, until the wound is healed, before allowing nonweight-bearing active range of motion (**Fig. 5**). Surgical dressings remain intact for 10-14 days and are then seen in the office. It is not uncommon to replace the posterior splint for an additional week before suture removal and ROM is allowed if the wound is not properly healed. If other procedures are performed the surgeon may appropriately postpone this "early" ROM.

Deep venous thrombosis prophylaxis and antibiotic prophylaxis is controversial and beyond the scope of this chapter. Many institutions have protocols that can be followed. The surgeon is obligated to investigate these issues and have a rational approach and support for the chosen treatment.

Casting and orthoses must be monitored by the surgeon as well. Many off-the-shelf products do not fit properly and can have devastating ramifications. It is recommended that walking boots be fit by the surgeon or an experienced staff member with a thorough explanation of the parameters for proper wear. An example of how quickly a problem can occur is the case of a 76-year-old patient, 20 days S/P TAA, doing well in the rehabilitation unit with a posterior splint. The incisions were healed, and a cam walker was ordered. Unfortunately, the regular orthotist was not available and the boot was placed by an inexperienced orthotist. The patient complained of pain from the time the boot was placed, but the boot was not removed. The physician was called 3 days later, and the boot was removed. Dressings had been applied improperly and the anterior ankle strap was very tight, resulting in full thickness pressure necrosis underneath the strap (**Fig. 6**A). Irrigation and debridement was unsuccessful and the patient underwent a BKA (**Fig. 6**B and C). This devastating outcome could have been prevented with close and appropriate postop monitoring. This type of complication is avoidable and highlights the importance of using experienced allied providers for all patients undergoing TAA.

Weight bearing is typically allowed at 6 weeks. This period allows for bony ingrowth along the implant–bone interface. Serial radiographs to monitor bony healing and

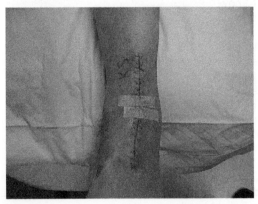

Fig. 5. This photo was taken 2-weeks postop TAA. The patient has been immobilized up to this point. Aggressive ROM may now be started because the wound has healed appropriately.

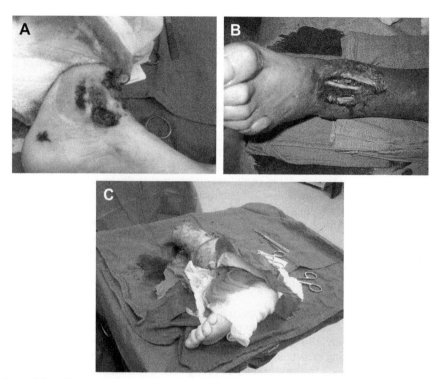

Fig. 6. (*A*) Patient with full thickness necrosis after inappropriate application of walking boot. (*B*) After debridement, notice exposed implant. (*C*) Implant removed, limb not viable, BKA performed.

clinical examination will determine the exact time to weight bear. This may be prolonged in patients who are elderly or who have DM or rheumatoid arthritis.

Complications

Common complications that require management or revision of TAA are as follows (reported rates, if known, are in parentheses): delayed wound healing (superficial 4%–17%), deep periprosthetic infection (0.5–3.5%), sensory deficits (10–21%), CRPS (0–4.3%), periprosthetic fracture, subsidence, malalignment, prosthesis loosening, syndesmotic nonunion, polyethelene failure, osteolysis, impingement, tendon injury, and stiffness.[13,27–29]

Complications arise from three main categories: (1) inappropriate patient selection, (2) surgeon inexperience and (3) surgeon error. These can largely be avoided by critical patient selection and proper surgeon training. I am often asked, "How are the total ankle implants doing?" This is a reasonable question in light of the fact that we must continue to improve upon the techniques and instrumentation. However, a more valid and appropriate question is, "How are the surgeons who are implanting total ankles doing?" Improvement in both aspects will continue to improve outcomes.

Deep periprosthetic infections (DPI) can be devastating. Early recognition and aggressive treatment is the key to salvaging the limb. Wound complications can be classified as either minor superficial infections presenting with superficial wound breakdown and edge necrosis, or as major wound complications that include deep infections that penetrate the deep fascial layer and subsequently the implant.[28,30]

Schuberth,[23] in his review of his first 50 Agility TAAs, reported a 20% incidence of wound complications. He found wound complications to be a consistent problem independent of surgeon experience. In contrast, Myerson[28] found a decrease in wound complications that correlated with surgeon experience. Ninety percent of his infections were classified as superficial and resolved with aggressive local wound care; one required flap coverage, and was therefore classified as a major complication requiring an antibiotic spacer and talar revision. They observed that all wound complications occurred in the same anatomic location, namely the anterior incision just superior to the joint line.

Buechel and colleagues[24] reported wound problems as the most common complication with a comparable rate of 17.4% in their 20-year review of 40 patients. They also commented on the inevitable complication inherent to the local anatomy.

A more recent article again found little correlation between surgeon experience and wound complications.[25] Evaluation of two groups consisting of 25 primary TAA produced a 12% wound complication rate. Four of the six complications resolved with topical dressing changes. Two required skin grafting and one lead to a major complication requiring an antibiotic spacer and revision total ankle replacement. The investigators attributed the lack of major wound complications to adequate incisions, limited subcutaneous dissection, judicious use of self-retaining retractors, and limited plantar flexion for 3 weeks.

Superficial infections can usually be managed conservatively by the surgeon with local wound care and/or negative pressure devices. Too often, practitioners not familiar with TAA turn a minor wound problem into a major problem by excessive probing and swabbing or overaggressive debridement, thus exposing the implant.

Deep periprosthetic infections should be recognized and treated quickly. Oral or IV antibiotics are not sufficient once a deep periprosthetic infection is diagnosed. Salvage in the face of DPI is typically a two-stage procedure. Debridement of nonvascular tissue along with deep tissue cultures is necessary, usually requiring removal of the implant. Debridement should be aggressive and will include removal of capsule, scar, and devitalized bone, followed by placement of an antibiotic cement spacer (**Fig. 7A-D**) . The cement spacer allows for high concentrations of local antibiotics and maintains length for future revision. I have been able to salvage some DPIs without implant removal using inflow/outflow irrigation and polyethelene exchange in a well-incorporated implant. This is accomplished with 5 days of keramycin saline inflow and active suction outflow.

Culture-specific IV antibiotics are administered and, in conjunction with cement spacer exchange, repeated debridements are repeated as necessary. Occasionally a soft tissue flap may be needed. A plastic surgeon can be valuable in assisting with soft tissue coverage; however, it is vital that the TAA surgeon remains directly involved in the care of the patient in order to prevent overly aggressive debridements and unnecessary exposure of the implant. During the convalescent phase, the wound should be monitored closely. Laboratory markers, including the erythrocyte sedimentation rate (ESR) and C-reactive protein (CRP), are followed to evaluate treatment.[31] Definitive revision of any kind should be delayed until resolution of infection is obtained clinically and by normalization of ESR and CRP. Final confirmation is best achieved with a deep aspiration culture and a bone biopsy.

If reimplantation is not possible, a conversion to an arthrodesis is possible. In some cases, fresh-frozen femoral head allograft is an option, but with a recent history of infection, I prefer autogenous iliac crest (**Fig. 8**).

Sensory deficits and nerve damage can occur due to laceration or traction injury from the surgical exposure. Every nerve crossing the ankle is at risk with TAA. The

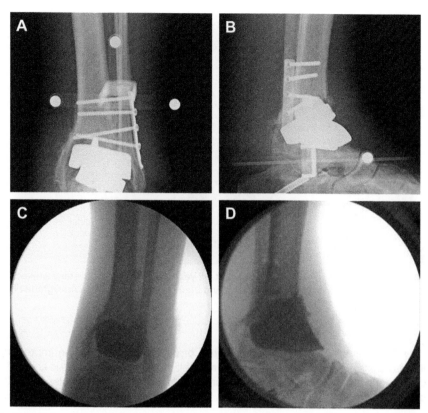

Fig. 7. Sixty-four-year-old male 6-months postop from TAA with infection from remote site seeded into TAA. (*A, B*) Anteroposterior (AP) and lateral radiographs showing anterior subsidence of the tibial component along with periprosthetic loosening. (*C, D*) Three-weeks postop after explantation with antibiotic-impregnated bone cement. Usually I re-implant patients with a TAA when the infection is resolved; however, in this patient a conversion to a fusion was recommended due to significant bone loss.

most common injury is to the superficial peroneal nerve crossing at the anterior ankle (**Fig. 4**A). Some patients have a branch of the superficial peroneal nerve that is directly anterior to the ankle joint. In this case, it is better to sharply resect the nerve away from the incision line rather than to risk an almost certain traction injury. Further into this same dissection plane, the deep peroneal nerve is also at risk. The tibial nerve and vessels are in the posterior medial portion of the bone resection. Posterior plunging of the saw blade can damage these structures (**Fig. 4**G) The sural and superficial peroneal nerves are at risk from the lateral incision where a plate is placed for syndesmotic arthrodesis in the agility system. The saphenous nerve can be damaged by the stab incision at the medial neck of the talus for external fixation pin placement (**Fig. 4**B).

Periprosthetic fractures present as either early or late complications. Regardless of the timing, both are usually the result of surgeon error. Early fractures are usually the result of surgeon error by commission. For instance, the posterior aspect of the distal tibia is tightly bound by strong capsular attachments and can be very difficult to remove during bone resection. Care and patience must be exercised during this portion of the procedure to prevent any pressure or torque on the fragile malleoli (**Fig. 9**). Late

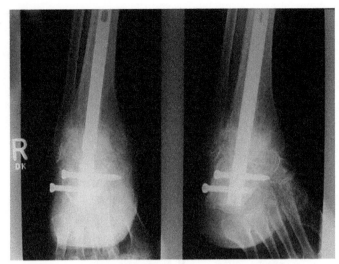

Fig. 8. AP and mortise radiographs of a patient 2.5 years postop with a two-stage conversion of TAA to arthrodesis. Autogenous iliac crest was used on end along with a retrograde tibial nail.

fractures are usually the result from an error of omission leading to an improperly balanced ankle. For example, a late medial malleolar fracture often occurs in an uncorrected valgus ankle because of the excessive pull from the deltoid complex (**Fig. 10**). **Fig. 11** shows the same patient as in **Fig. 10**, nine months status postfixation. This

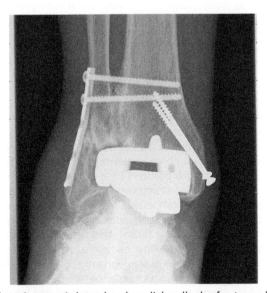

Fig. 9. Patient with an iatrogenic lateral and medial malleolar fractures due to overaggressive bone resection. The lateral malleolous has gone on to nonunion. Note periprosthetic lucency laterally along the tibial component.

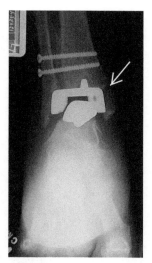

Fig.10. Arrow is pointing to an avulsion medial malleolar fracture caused by excessive valgus in the ankle.

patient did not have the valgus corrected and the medial malleolous fractured again in just 9 months. In this scenario, revision must include correcting the underlying valgus moment in addition to the fracture.

Subsidence of the prosthetic components can also occur. One advantage of the Agility system is that it incorporates the tibial and fibular cortical bone as well as a syndesmotic arthrodesis for tibial component support (**Fig. 12**). The Inbone has a large, porous, coated stem that provides support to the tibial component (**Fig. 13**). The Salto talaris ankle offers less total bone resection, resecting less bone results in the implant

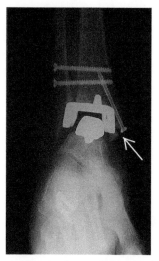

Fig. 11. In the same patient as in **Fig. 10**, the medial malleolar fracture was repaired and healed, but has now recurred (*arrow*) due to the lack of correction of the valgus moment about the ankle.

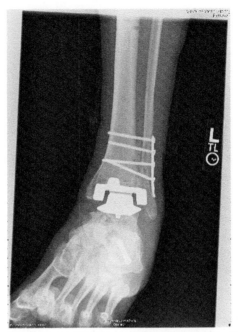

Fig. 12. One-year status post-TAA. Note how the implant rests laterally on cortical bone of both the tibia and fibula as well as a solid syndesmotic arthrodesis.

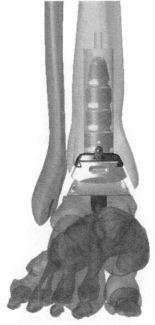

Fig. 13. Schematic of the Inbone TAA. Note the stem in the tibial canal providing support to the tibial component.

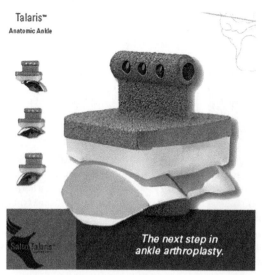

Fig. 14. The Salto Talaris TAA. Minimal bone resection allows the Salto to rest on stronger distal tibial bone. It also allows the talus to dictate the "sweet spot" of the final position of the tibial component.

resting on stronger bone (**Fig. 14**). Distal tibial bone rapidly loses strength as resection is brought more proximal. The Agility has had some complications with talar subsidence. The early designs, with a very narrow talar component, were problematic. The new Agility LP (low profile) has a significantly larger talar component covering most if not all of the cut surface of talus, and has decreased the incidence of talar subsidence (**Fig. 15**). The Tournier and Inbone ankle have a resurfacing talar component and subsidence is rare.

Prosthetic loosening is caused by failure of proper bony ingrowth or disruption of bony ingrowth called "aseptic loosening." Aseptic loosening is usually accompanied by pain and a dark halo around the loose component due to insufficient bony ingrowth (**Fig. 16**A and B). These implants need revision to decrease pain and to prevent bone

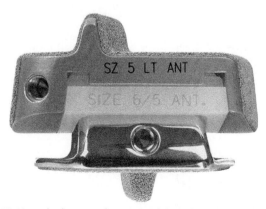

Fig. 15. The Agility LP. Note the large surface area of the talar component. This is designed to resist talar subsidence (Copyright DePuy Orthopaedics, Inc. Warsaw, IN; with permission).

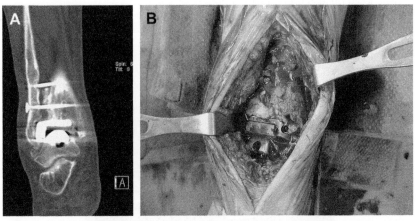

Fig.16. (*A*) Patient with lateral tibial subsidence; notice the syndesmotic nonunion. (*B*) After removal of loose tibial component and re-implantation with cement fixation of the tibia and re-fusion of the syndesmosis.

loss and deformity. Septic loosening is caused by infection and is an emergent situation to remove the implant. (Please see the section on deep periprosthetic infections, above.)

Osteolysis is caused from microscopic debris causing a macrophage-mediated cystic response in the bone. Osteolysis can be seen on radiographs as lucent areas in the tibia, talus, or fibula. Saltzman and colleagues[32,33] described periprosthetic lucencies and lysis. A lucency was defined as a radiolucent line 2 mm wide, and lysis was defined as a radiolucent area of greater than 2 mm. Mechanical lysis occurs early after implantation along the fibular border of the Agility implant and usually ceases as bony ingrowth matures (**Fig. 17**). In contrast to mechanical lysis is expansile lysis,

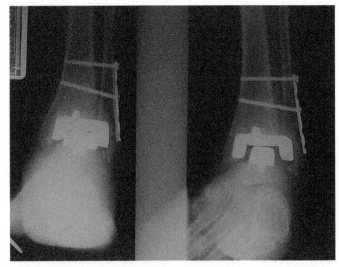

Fig. 17. Mechanical osteolysis between the tibial component and the fibula.

which usually occurs later (3–5 years) and is more progressive, in many cases requiring evacuation and bone grafting to prevent weakening of the bone and possible pathologic fracture (**Fig. 18**).[34]

Revision and Complicated Total Ankle Arthroplasty

When failures occur, they can be revised in most cases. The most common reasons for major revision are subsidence and surgeon error in implantation.[17] Infection is devastating in TAA: although revision is possible, it is fraught with complications and pitfalls (see above discussion of deep periprosthetic infections).

Subsidence can be caused from soft bone, overly aggressive bone resection, improper prosthesis placement, sepsis, and too small of an implant. If tibial subsidence occurs in the Agility implant, it is usually secondary to a nonunion of the syndesmosis. Revision is performed if symptomatic or progressive and consists of re-fusion of the syndesmosis and realigning the tibial component either with cement or autogenous bone graft (**Fig. 16**A and B). Talar subsidence can be even more challenging. Often, as the talar component subsides, it will fracture into or even rest in the subtalar joint. Revision components can be made to tackle this difficult situation and fuse the subtalar joint simultaneously (**Fig. 19**).

As arthritis progresses, the joint space is obliterated and supporting medial and lateral ligaments become attenuated. Ligamentous structures can also be attenuated by repeated mechanical injury in the disease process. One of the main goals of TAA is to tension the joint, meaning to bring the joint back out to length so that the supporting soft tissue structures can function in a stabilizing manner once again. Failure to achieve proper tension produces a loose joint prone to frontal plane instability. These joints are usually revised due to pain and deformity.

Patients who have a previous triple arthrodesis with progressive ankle arthrosis can be ideal candidates for TAA, and avoid a pantalar arthrodesis. However, the surgeon must be certain that a malpositioned triple is not the cause of the ankle arthrosis. A malpositioned triple will cause the TAA to fail as well. In some instances, an ankle arthrodesis can be taken down and TAA performed in order to avoid a pantalar arthrodesis, or in cases of ankle fusion mal- or nonunions. A patient had a painful nonunion taken down and an Agility TAA implanted 3 years ago. His ankle ROM is 6

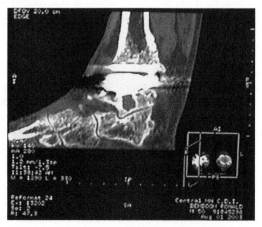

Fig. 18. Expansile lysis seen on CT inferior to the talar component.

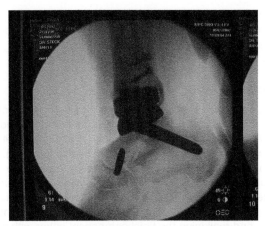

Fig. 19. An Agility TAA with a custom stemmed talar component to salvage a previously subsided talar component into the subtalar joint.

degrees of dorsiflexion and 18 degrees of plantarflexion. He states he would do it again.

In my experience with 400 Agility TAA 1–6 year follow-up, I have had six (1.5%) DPIs requiring implant removal: three were re-implanted with an Agility TAA, one elected to keep a cement spacer, one went on to a fusion at the patients request, and one needed a BKA. Patient satisfaction is over 90%. Major complication (necessitating metal implant revision) rate is 8% (32 patients). One patient total required a BKA. The rate of minor complication, requiring any take back to the OR for any reason related to the TAA or superficial infection not involving the implant, is14% (56 patients).

SUMMARY

TAA has a steep learning curve and is a technically demanding procedure that can be intensified when adding a complicating factor, such as a patient who has DM or multiple relative contraindications. The surgical technique is where the learning curve is keenly felt. However, with meticulous patient selection, lack of neuropathy and vascular disease, as well as good surgeon training and a well-thought out implant, positive results can be obtained that are challenging the gold standard of fusion.

ACKNOWLEDGMENTS

I would like to thank Dr. Randall Gall for cementing in me a love for foot and ankle surgery and how to think critically; Dr. Frank Alvine for his friendship and the truly amazing three years of working with a true master surgeon; he taught me so much about total ankle replacement, but so much more about life; Gundersen Lutheran Medical Center in Lacrosse, Wisc., for providing me with a solid academic foundation; and most of all my family, for all they help me with and their sacrifices in my professional endeavors.

REFERENCES

1. Mazur JM, Schwartz E, Simon SR. Ankle arthrodesis: long-term follow-up with gait analysis. J Bone Joint Surg Am 1979;61:964–75.

2. Takakura Y, Tanaka Y, Sugimoto K, et al. Long-term results of arthrodesis for oste-oarthritis of the ankle. Clin Orthop 1999;361:178–85.
3. Fuchs S, Sandmann C, Skwara A, et al. Quality of life 20 years after arthrodesis of the ankle. A study of adjacent joints. J Bone Joint Surg Br 2003;85:994–8.
4. Doets HC, Van Middelkoop M, Houdijk H, Nelissen RGHH, Veeger HEJ. Gait analysis after total ankle arthroplasty: a comparative study with a normal control group. Presented at the Annual Meeting of the American Academy of Orthopaedic Surgeons. Washington, DC, Feb 23–27, 2005.
5. Coester LM, Saltzman CL, Leupold J, et al. Long-term results following ankle arthrodesis for post-traumatic arthritis. J Bone Joint Surg Am 2001;83:219–28.
6. McGuire MR, Kyle RF, Gustilo RB, et al. Comparative analysis of ankle arthroplasty versus ankle arthrodesis. Clin Orthop 1998;226:174–81.
7. Kitaoka HB, Claridge RJ. Ankle replacement arthroplasty. In: Morrey BF, editor. Joint replacement arthroplasty. edition 3. Philadelphia, PA: Churchill-Livingston; 2003. p. 1133–50.
8. Coughlin MJ. The Scandinavian total ankle replacement prosthesis. Instr Course Lect 2002;51:135–42.
9. Kitaoka HB, Patzer GL. Clinical results of the Mayo Total Ankle Arthroplasty. J Bone Joint Surg 1996;78(A):1658–64.
10. Bolton-Maggs BG, Sudlow RA, Freeman MAR. Total ankle arthroplasty: a long-term review of the London hospital experience. J Bone Joint Surg 1985;67B(5):785–90.
11. Stauffer RN. Salvage of painful total ankle arthroplasty. Clin Orthop 1982;October(170):184–8.
12. Takakura Y, Tanaka Y, Sugimoto K, et al. Ankle arthroplasty: a comparative study of cemented metal and uncemented ceramic prostheses. Clin Orthop Relat Res 1990;252:209–16.
13. Pyevich MT, Saltzman CL, Callaghan JJ, et al. Total ankle arthroplasty: a unique design. Two-to twelve-year follow-up. J Bone Joint Surg Am 1998;80:1410–20.
14. Spirt AA, Assal M, Hansen ST Jr. Complications and failure after total ankle arthroplasty. J Bone Joint Surg Am 2004;86A:1172–8.
15. Kitaoka HB, Patzer GL, Ilstrup DM, et al. Survivorship analysis of the Mayo Total Ankle Arthroplasty. J Bone Joint Surg Am 1994;76:974–9.
16. Kofoed H, Lundberg-Jensen A. Ankle arthroplasty in patients younger and older than 50 years: a prospective series with long-term follow-up. Foot Ankle 1999;20:501–6.
17. Haddad SL, Coetzee JC, Estok R, et al. Intermediate and long-term outcomes of total ankle arthroplasty and ankle arthrodesis: a systematic review of the literature. J Bone Joint Surg Am 2007;89:1899–905.
18. Crosby CT, Mares AK. Skin antisepsis: past, present, and future. J Vasc Access 2000;6(1):26–31.
19. Knupp M, Valderrabano V, Hintermann B. Anatomical and biomechanical aspects of total ankle replacement. Orthopade 2006;35(5):489–94.
20. Henricson A, Skoog A, Carlsson A. The Swedish ankle arthroplasty register: an analysis of 531 arthroplasties between 1993 and 2005. Acta Orthop 2007;78(5):569–74.
21. Haskell A, Mann RA. Perioperative complication rate of total ankle replacement is reduced by surgeon experience. Foot Ankle Int 2004;25:789–93.
22. Saltzman CL, Amendola A, Anderson R, et al. Surgeon training and complications in total ankle arthroplasty. Foot Ankle Int 2003;24(6):514–8.

23. Schuberth JM, Patel S, Zarutsky E. Perioperative complications of the agility total ankle replacement in 50 initial consecutive cases. J Foot Ankle Surg 2006;45: 139–46.
24. Beuchel FF, Pappas MJ, Iorio LJ. New Jersey low contact stress total ankle replacement: biomechanical rationale and review of 23 cementless cases. Foot Ankle 1988;8:279–90.
25. Lee KB, Cho SG, Hur CI, et al. Perioperative complications of HINTEGRA total ankle replacement: our initial 50 cases. Foot Ankle Int 2008;29(10):978–84.
26. Soohoo NF, Kominski G. Cost-effectiveness analysis of total ankle arthroplasty. J Bone Joint Surg Am 2004;86-A(11):2446–55.
27. Garcia R, Mulberry G, Brady A, et al. Comparison of ChloraPrep and Betadine as preoperative skin preparation antiseptics. Poster presented at 40th Annual Meeting of the Infectious Disease Society of America; Chicago, October 25, 2002.
28. Myerson MS, Mroczek K. Perioperative complications of total ankle arthroplasty. Foot Ankle Int 2003;24(1):17–21.
29. Conti SF, Wong YS. Complications of total ankle arthroplasty. Clin Orthop 2001; 391(1):105–14.
30. Havid I, Rasmussen O, Jensen NC, et al. Trabecular bone strength profiles at the ankle joint. Clin Orthop 1985;October(199):306–12.
31. Khan MH, Smith PN, Rao N, et al. Serum C-reactive protein levels correlate with clinical response in patients treated with antibiotics for wound infections after spinal surgery. Spine J 2006;6(3):311–5.
32. Saltzman CL. Total ankle arthroplasty: state of the art. Instr Course Lect 1999;48: 263–8.
33. Buechel FF Sr, Pappas MJ, Buechel FF Jr. Twenty-year evaluation of cementless mobile-bearing total ankle replacements. Clin Orthop 2004;424:19–26.
34. Knecht SI, Estin M, Callaghan JJ, et al. The Agility total ankle arthroplasty. J Bone Joint Surg Am 2004;86:1161–71.

Current Concepts and Techniques
in Foot and Ankle Surgery

Combined Medial Displacement Calcaneal Osteotomy, Subtalar Joint Arthrodesis, and Ankle Arthrodiastasis for End-Stage Posterior Tibial Tendon Dysfunction

John J. Stapleton, DPM[a,b], Ronald Belczyk, DPM[c],
Thomas Zgonis, DPM, FACFAS[c,]*, Vasilios D. Polyzois, MD, PhD[d]

KEYWORDS

- Posterior tibial tendon dysfunction • Calcaneal osteotomy
- Subtalar joint arthrodesis • Ankle arthrodiastasis
- External fixation • Taylor spatial frame

Pantalar or tibiotalocalcaneal (TTC) arthrodesis is the standard treatment for end-stage posterior tibial tendon dysfunction (PTTD) with severe ankle joint arthrosis and after failure of conservative management. Stage 4 PTTD commonly causes painful joint arthrosis about the rearfoot and ankle with a rigid pes planovalgus deformity. The combination of deformity, pain, and loss of motion associated with end-stage PTTD makes surgical management a challenging problem. Currently, surgical treatment options for stage 4 PTTD are limited to rearfoot joint fusions combined with ankle arthrodesis or endoprosthesis. The literature supports a pantalar or TTC arthrodesis despite the potential complications associated with either procedure. Including an ankle arthrodesis may be suitable for older, inactive, or sedentary patients. Younger patients affected with severe deformity and joint arthrosis from neglected or undiagnosed end-stage PTTD with ankle joint involvement may benefit from a joint salvage procedure. Unfortunately, ankle endoprosthesis has had limited success in the

[a] VSAS Orthopaedics, Allentown, PA, USA
[b] Department of Surgery, Penn State College of Medicine, Hershey, PA, USA
[c] Division of Podiatric Medicine and Surgery, Department of Orthopaedics, The University of Texas Health Science Center at San Antonio, 7703 Floyd Curl Drive/MCS 7776, San Antonio, TX 78229, USA
[d] Orthopaedic Traumatology, KAT General Hospital, Athens, Greece
* Corresponding author.
E-mail address: zgonis@uthscsa.edu (T. Zgonis).

Clin Podiatr Med Surg 26 (2009) 325–333
doi:10.1016/j.cpm.2009.01.001
0891-8422/09/$ – see front matter © 2009 Elsevier Inc. All rights reserved.

younger and active patient population with painful ankle arthrosis, and many surgeons advise its use be limited to patients who have light physical demands. Ankle joint distraction (arthrodiastasis) offers another treatment option to delay or prevent the need for an ankle arthrodesis. This article discusses a novel technique not yet reported in the scientific literature that incorporates an ankle arthrodiastasis combined with a medial displacement calcaneal osteotomy (MDCO) and a subtalar joint arthrodesis for end-stage PTTD.

HISTORICAL PERSPECTIVE

Surgical management of stage 4 PTTD in young and otherwise active patients is a challenge. In this population, stage 4 PTTD usually is the result of a neglected or misdiagnosed posterior tibial tendon tear or rupture. Pantalar and TTC arthrodesis procedures have been associated with high rates of complications including nonunion in up to 60% and postoperative infection in up to 25%.[1,2] Different techniques for a pantalar and TTC arthrodesis have been described using various forms of internal and external fixation.[1-3] Despite advances in internal and external fixation along with the improved fusion rates, a pantalar or TTC arthrodesis is considered a salvage procedure and used cautiously in primary reconstructive cases.[1-3] A successful pantalar or TTC fusion can alleviate pain and correct deformity at the expense of joint motion.[4] Loss of joint motion about the rearfoot and ankle causes persistent alterations in gait that may lead to severe restriction of activity.[5,6] It also may lead to increased stress and deterioration of adjoining joints by ipsilateral or contralateral overloading or compensation.[5,6]

Other joint-sparing procedures have incorporated the use of deltoid ligament reconstructive procedures and, at times, lateral ankle stabilization procedures combined with rearfoot fusions to correct alignment of the ankle mortise.[7] These procedures are beneficial for achieving deformity correction but offer little for the management of painful ankle arthrosis. In theory, combining realignment of the rearfoot with an ankle arthrodiastasis can preserve motion to prevent major alterations in gait while avoiding the complications commonly associated with an ankle arthrodesis.[8]

The rationale behind the authors' technique is performing a MDCO to realign the weight-bearing forces with the lower leg. In addition, if the subtalar joint is associated with an end-stage arthrosis, a subtalar joint arthrodesis is selected to eliminate pain and prevent further collapse from the dysfunctional posterior tibial tendon. Ankle arthrodiastasis in conjunction with an open ankle arthrotomy is performed simultaneously to prevent and delay the need for an ankle arthrodesis or endoprosthesis.[8] Ankle arthrodiastasis can be performed as an alternative to ankle arthrodesis to relieve pain and improve joint function.[8-18] Joint distraction, using a circular external fixation frame that bridges the ankle joint, is a fairly new approach in the treatment of severe ankle joint arthrosis. A tension wire circular external fixation device allows surgeons the ability to distract the surrounding soft tissues of a stiff joint, permit weight bearing, reduce the mechanical stress across a joint, and apply intermittent intra-articular fluid pressures across a joint through axial loading and unloading.[8-18] Research on osteoarthritic cartilage has shown that intermittent hydrostatic pressures applied in the absence of mechanical stress could result in reparative activity by chondrocytes through the production of proteoglycans.[9-18]

Joint distraction via external fixation for the treatment of severe osteoarthritis in young patients was first described in 1994 for the hip.[19] In 1995 van Valburg and colleagues[17] published the results of a retrospective study in a preliminary report that included 11 patients, with a mean age of 35 ± 13 years, in which joint distraction was used as an alternative to ankle arthrodesis to treat posttraumatic arthrosis of the ankle. They concluded that at an average of 20 months (9–60) postoperatively short-term joint distraction can be used to delay arthrodesis because none of the patients had proceeded to an ankle arthrodesis. Range of motion improved in 55% of these patients. All 11 patients had less pain and five patients had no pain.[17] In 1999, van Valburg and colleagues[12] published the data from the first prospective study on ankle joint distraction with a 2-year follow-up. The conclusion confirmed the previous findings in their retrospective study supporting the notion that joint distraction can delay the need for ankle arthrodesis in the presence of severe ankle arthrosis.[12] They found that more than two thirds of the patients improved significantly, as shown by physical examination, functional ability questionnaires, and pain scale.[12] The results were progressive in the second year postoperatively.[12] In 2002 Marijnissen and colleagues[15] published the results of an open prospective study of 57 patients, average age 44 years, treated with joint distraction as an alternative to ankle arthrodesis. Clinical benefit was apparent in three fourths of the 57 patients. Most importantly, the clinical benefit of joint distraction increased over time postoperatively as opposed to ankle and pantalar arthrodesis.[15]

Ankle joint arthrodiastasis is a joint-sparing procedure and the authors have combined this technique with simultaneous rearfoot realignment and arthrodesis procedures to manage end-stage PTTD successfully. This article describes the technique of ankle arthrodiastasis using the Taylor spatial frame (TSF).

SURGICAL TECHNIQUE

The surgical technique of combined MDCO, subtalar joint arthrodesis, and ankle arthrodiastasis begins with a patient under general, spinal, or regional anesthesia when indicated. The lower extremity should be directly supine avoiding any internal or external rotation. In addition, it is imperative to have the lower extremity prepped and draped above the knee joint and allow room for the placement of the thigh tourniquet. This enables a surgeon the ability to evaluate the alignment of the foot, ankle, and lower leg. Any concomitant soft tissue procedures, such as an Achilles tendon lengthening or gastrocnemius recession, are performed initially.

In the authors' case (**Fig. 1**), a percutaneous triple hemisection of the Achilles tendon for lengthening was performed first followed by an oblique lateral incision just posterior to the peroneal tendons for the MDCO. The lateral incision was fashioned in the same direction as the oblique calcaneal osteotomy. The sural nerve and vascular structures were identified and retracted posteriorly and the incision then was carried down to the lateral surface of the calcaneus. Minimal reflection of the periosteum was performed to allow for the placement of the osteotomy. Hohmann retractors were placed to identify the superior and inferior borders of the calcaneal osteotomy. A combination of a powered sagittal saw with a wide blade and an osteotome then was used to perform the osteotomy. The technique involved cupping the heel with the contralateral hand so the depth of the blade and control of the heel were maintained while performing the osteotomy. The osteotomy was completed with an osteotome and a smooth lamina spreader placed into the osteotomy site and distracted to stretch the tissues on the medial aspect of the heel and to facilitate the medial displacement of the calcaneus. The tuberosity of the calcaneus then was translated approximately 10 to 12 mm and held provisionally with two guide wires. The osteotomy can be secured with a cannulated screw over a guide wire or a step-off staple, as used in this case. It is imperative to confirm the position of the osteotomy by lateral and calcaneal axial views under intraoperative fluoroscopy.

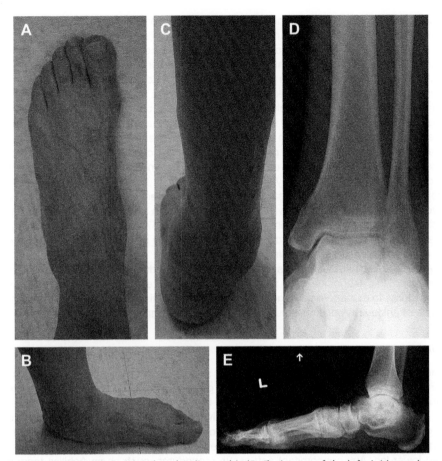

Fig. 1. Preoperative clinical (*A–C*) and radiographic (*D–E*) pictures of the left rigid pes plano-valgus deformity and concomitant ankle arthrosis. Intraoperative picture showing the incision and calcaneal osteotomy placement (*F*) followed by use of internal fixation (*G*). Medial approach for the subtalar joint arthrodesis (*H*) or tendon transfer if necessary and after the MDCO is performed. Intraoperative anteroposterior (*I*) and lateral (*J*) fluoroscopy imaging showing the ankle arthrodiastasis procedure with use of a TSF. A calcaneal axial imaging showing the calcaneal osteotomy fixation and alignment (*K*). Postoperative pictures (*L, M*) of the external fixator at 4 weeks' follow-up. Final clinical (*N–P*) and radiographic pictures (*Q, R*) at 2 years' follow-up and without any related symptoms.

Overhang of the lateral wall of the calcaneus should be tamped down to prevent soft tissue irritation postoperatively.

Attention then is directed to the medial aspect of the foot for the subtalar joint arthrodesis. In the authors' case, a medial incision was used to perform the subtalar joint arthrodesis to further prevent skin necrosis laterally given the severity of the valgus deformity while allowing repair of the spring ligament and posterior tibial tendon. It is the authors' opinion that when a calcaneal valgus deformity exceeds 25° of the rearfoot deformity, a medial incision may be used when an acute correction is performed to prevent wound dehiscence or necrosis at the lateral aspect of the foot. A 5-cm curvilinear incision is placed just above the sustentaculum tali, extending just distal to the navicular tuberosity if the flexor digitorum longus (FDL) is harvested for

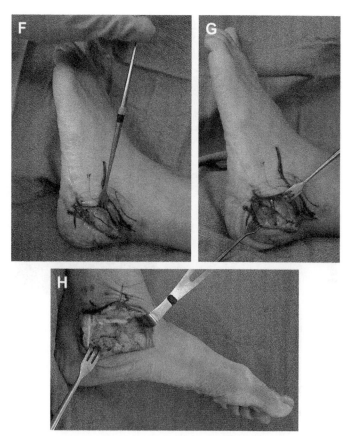

Fig. 1. (*continued*)

a tendon transfer. After the medial incision is made, the flexor retinaculum is incised and the sheaths of the posterior tibial and FDL tendons are identified along with the neurovascular bundle, which is mobilized and retracted with vessel loupes to minimize traumatic injury. Dissection then is carried down full thickness just superior to the sustentaculum tali. The middle facet is identified with a curved osteotome that is advanced into the posterior facet. A curved elevator is passed around the posterior aspect of the subtalar joint while a lamina spreader is placed into the floor of the sinus tarsi. Most often, the contents of the sinus tarsi have to be resected to facilitate distraction and exposure of the subtalar joint. Any remaining articular cartilage is meticulously removed with an osteotome or a curved curette to maintain the contour of the joint. The area is irrigated copiously to ensure that all debris is removed from the prepared joints and that the subchondral plate is drilled to stimulate vascular ingrowth in preparation for the arthrodesis. After appropriate positioning, the arthrodesis site can be stabilized temporarily with a Steinmann pin until the external fixator is applied. Internal fixation also may be used to fixate the subtalar joint arthrodesis site and the external fixator is applied only to achieve distraction across the ankle joint.

The posterior tibial tendon can be repaired or advanced if good muscle excursion exists or it is excised and the FDL tendon is transferred through a drill hole placed into the navicular. An alternative is to use the posterior tibial tendon for reconstruction of the deltoid ligament if needed and if a FDL transfer is performed.

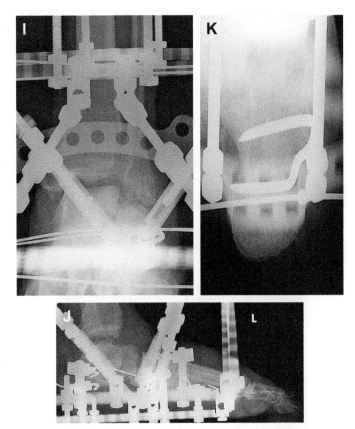

Fig. 1. (*continued*)

Attention then is directed to the anterior aspect of the ankle joint. In the presence of an anterior ankle joint impingement or osseous spurring noted to the anterior distal tibia or talus, an arthroscopic or open ankle arthrotomy is performed. At that time, excision of hypertrophic and hemorrhagic synovium and subchondral drilling or micro-fracture of any osteochondral defects of the ankle joint can be performed. After closure of the wounds, the pneumatic thigh tourniquet is released. The prebuilt multi-plane circular external fixator that consists of two tibia rings and a footplate is posi-tioned to the lower extremity and held with towels underneath the posterior aspect of the heel and lower leg. The construct of the external fixator consists of two or three smooth wires or half pins attached to each tibia ring, opposing olive wires into the calcaneus, and a talar and a midfoot wire. Each wire is placed in anatomic safe zones and tensioned appropriately. Typical tension of wires in the tibia ranges from 110 to 130 kg and wires in the foot range from 50 to 90 kg. The smooth wire through the talus is placed into the body of the talus in line with the bisection of the medial and lateral malleolus. After the wire is placed into the talus, it is pulled proximal and inferior to attach to the footplate. This bent wire is tensioned manually to compress across the subtalar joint.

Distraction is performed at the ankle joint by turning and adjusting the struts on the TSF between the distal tibia ring and the footplate to obtain 8 to 10 mm of symmetric ankle joint distraction. Distraction across the ankle joint is confirmed through

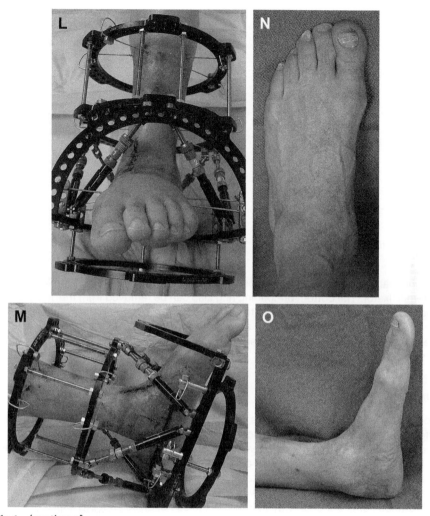

Fig. 1. (*continued*)

intraoperative fluoroscopy imaging. One of the advantages of using the TSF in the ankle arthrodiastasis procedure is its accuracy and easier application in the operating field. It also allows a surgeon to adjust for any postoperative corrections in an efficient way.

POSTOPERATIVE MANAGEMENT

Postoperatively, patients are admitted to a hospital for pain, edema control, observation, and physical therapy for upper and lower extremity strengthening. Patient neurovascular status is checked routinely every 4 to 6 hours for the first 24 hours if a regional block was not used. Attention is paid to signs and symptoms of increased pain along the tarsal tunnel. If present, the amount of acute distraction is reduced and patients reassessed. If the pain is controlled better, gradual distraction is reapplied. Patients are non–weight bearing for the first 7 to 10 days for pain and edema control. At approximately 2 weeks and during the first postoperative visit, patients can begin

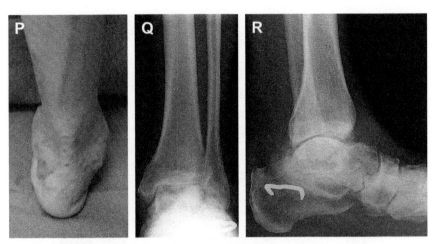

Fig. 1. (*continued*)

weight bearing as tolerated with a postoperative shoe attached to the footplate of the external fixator. The bottom off-loading ring also can be removed from the footplate if needed at that time. The circular external fixator is removed in approximately 8 to 10 weeks and patients progressed to a walking boot and physical therapy for 4 to 6 weeks. Patients can return to their normal activities between 4 and 6 months postoperatively.

SUMMARY

Combining an ankle arthrodiastasis with a MDCO and a subtalar joint arthrodesis offers surgeons a joint-sparing procedure for young and active patients who have end-stage PTTD and ankle joint involvement. An isolated subtalar joint arthrodesis or triple arthrodesis combined with an ankle arthrodiastasis is an option that can be used in certain case scenarios. Delaying the need for a joint destructive procedure through an ankle arthrodiastasis, however, may have a great impact in the near future, as advancements are underway to improve the use of ankle endoprosthesis.

REFERENCES

1. Goebel M, Gerdesmeyer L, Muckley T, et al. Retrograde intramedullary nailing in tibiotalocalcaneal arthrodesis: a short-term, prospective study. J Foot Ankle Surg 2006;45(2):98–106.
2. Mendicino RW, Catanzariti AR, Saltrick KR, et al. Tibiotalocalcaneal arthrodesis with retrograde intramedullary nailing. J Foot Ankle Surg 2004;43(2):82–6.
3. Zgonis T, Jolly GP, Blume P. External fixation use in arthrodesis of the foot and ankle. Clin Podiatr Med Surg 2004;21(1):1–15.
4. Mandracchia VJ, Mandi DM, Nickles WA, et al. Pantalar arthrodesis. Clin Podiatr Med Surg 2004;21(3):461–70.
5. Buchner M, Sabo D. Ankle fusion attributable to posttraumatic arthrosis: a long-term followup of 48 patients. Clin Orthop Relat Res 2003;(406):155–64.
6. Boobbyer GN. The long-term results of ankle arthrodesis. Acta Orthop Scand 1981;52(1):107–10.

7. Bluman EM, Title CI, Myerson MS. Posterior tibial tendon rupture: a refined classification system. Foot Ankle Clin 2007;12(2):233–49, v.
8. Zgonis T, Stapleton JJ, Roukis TS. Use of circular external fixation for combined subtalar joint fusion and ankle distraction. Clin Podiatr Med Surg 2008;25(4): 745–53.
9. Buckwalter JA. Joint distraction for osteoarthritis. Lancet 1996;347(8997): 279–80, 3.
10. van Roermund PM, Lafeber FP. Joint distraction as treatment for ankle osteoarthritis. Instr Course Lect 1999;48:249–54.
11. Chiodo CP, McGarvey W. Joint distraction for the treatment of ankle osteoarthritis. Foot Ankle Clin 2004;9(3):541–53.
12. van Valburg AA, van Roermund PM, Marijnissen AC, et al. Joint distraction in treatment of osteoarthritis: a two-year follow-up of the ankle. Osteoarthr Cartil 1999;7(5):474–9.
13. van Roermund PM, Marijnissen AC, Lafeber FP. Joint distraction as an alternative for the treatment of osteoarthritis. Foot Ankle Clin 2002;7(3):515–27.
14. van Roermund PM, van Valburg AA, Duivemann E, et al. Function of stiff joints may be restored by Ilizarov joint distraction. Clin Orthop Relat Res 1998;(348): 220–7.
15. Marijnissen AC, Van Roermund PM, Van Melkebeek J, et al. Clinical benefit of joint distraction in the treatment of severe osteoarthritis of the ankle: proof of concept in an open prospective study and in a randomized controlled study. Arthritis Rheum 2002;46(11):2893–902.
16. Marijnissen AC, van Roermund PM, van Melkebeek J, et al. Clinical benefit of joint distraction in the treatment of ankle osteoarthritis. Foot Ankle Clin 2003;8(2): 335–46.
17. van Valburg AA, van Roermund PM, Lammens J, et al. Can Ilizarov joint distraction delay the need for an arthrodesis of the ankle? A preliminary report. J Bone Joint Surg Br 1995;77(5):720–5.
18. Paley D, Lamm BM. Ankle joint distraction. Foot Ankle Clin 2005;10(4):685–98.
19. Aldegheri R, Trivella G, Saleh M. Articulated distraction of the hip. Conservative surgery for arthritis in young patients. Clin Orthop Relat Res 1994;(301):94–101.

A Case Report of a Simultaneous Local Osteochondral Autografting and Ankle Arthrodiastasis for the Treatment of a Talar Dome Defect

Ronald Belczyk, DPM[a], John J. Stapleton, DPM[b,c],
Thomas Zgonis, DPM, FACFAS[a],*, Vasilios D. Polyzois, MD, PhD[d]

KEYWORDS

- Osteochondral talar defect • Talar cartilage repair
- Ankle arthritis • Ilizarov external fixation • Ankle arthrodiastasis

Talar osteochondral defects (OCDs) continue to be a challenge for treating physicians because they frequently are missed or diagnosed incorrectly, often resulting in severe degenerative arthritis of the ankle joint. In general, the impact of degenerative arthritis is significant, affecting more than 20 million Americans and costing the United States economy more than $60 billion per year.[1] More specifically, talar dome lesions alone account for 0.09% of all fractures and 1% of fractures involving the talus.[2] Common etiologies of talar OCDs include trauma, chronic ankle instability, and lower extremity deformity. Patients typically present with symptoms of joint pain, edema, limitation of motion, and locking of the ankle joint. Treatment goals of talar OCDs include the reduction of pain, preserving ankle joint motion, and limiting the progression of ankle osteoarthritis. Nonoperative management includes cast immobilization; life change modifications, such as converting to nonimpact exercises; weight loss; bracing; nonsteroidal anti-inflammatory medications; or corticosteroid injections. Larger talar

[a] Division of Podiatric Medicine and Surgery, Department of Orthopaedics, The University of Texas Health Science Center at San Antonio, 7703 Floyd Curl Drive/MCS 7776, San Antonio, TX 78229, USA
[b] Foot and Ankle Surgery, VSAS Orthopaedics, Allentown, PA, USA
[c] Department of Surgery, Penn State College of Medicine, Hershey, PA, USA
[d] Orthopaedic Traumatology, KAT General Hospital, Athens, Greece
* Corresponding author.
E-mail address: zgonis@uthscsa.edu (T. Zgonis).

Clin Podiatr Med Surg 26 (2009) 335–342
doi:10.1016/j.cpm.2009.01.002
0891-8422/09/$ – see front matter © 2009 Elsevier Inc. All rights reserved.

OCDs and defects associated with loose bodies within the joint usually are not amenable to conservative treatment and delaying surgical intervention can lead to further damage to viable surrounding cartilage. Surgical intervention becomes a viable option in the presence of larger OCDs associated with loose bodies or osteochondral lesions that have failed conservative treatment. Surgical methods vary according to surgeon preference or are based on staging according to the Berndt-Harty classification.[3] Some of the first-line surgical interventions include excision, excision with drilling or microfracture, arthroscopy, and retrograde drilling.[3] These methods, however, replace defects with fibrocartilage, which is inferior in durability and biomechanical properties. These techniques may be suitable for smaller lesions or as a first-line surgical treatment in larger defects before consideration of osteochondral autografts. Advanced methods include biologic repair and regeneration of cartilage using cultured or autologous chondrocytes, osteochondral grafts, periosteal flaps, perichondral grafts, and arthrodiastasis.[3]

The successful use of autologous osteochondral autograft in the knee has promoted the applicability in the ankle. Sammarco and Makwana presented their results in 12 patients who had osteochondral lesions of the talus treated with excision and local osteochondral autogenous grafting.[4] They believed that the talus was a viable source of cartilage and that the local harvesting of cartilage avoided two separate joint exposures, thereby minimizing the morbidity of using an asymptomatic joint as a donor site. This case report describes a unique technique for the treatment of large talar osteochondral lesions using a local osteochondral autograft combined with an ankle arthrodiastasis.

CASE REPORT

A 53-year-old man was referred to the authors' outpatient clinic with a severe pain to his left ankle joint. The patient had tried physical therapy stretching exercises, intra-articular steroid injections, and shoe modifications before his referral visit. Radiographs and MRI of the left ankle demonstrated a 20 × 5 × 8–mm osteochondral defect in the medial talar dome along with an overlying cartilage loss and a very small lateral lesion without any cartilage loss. After several discussions about his conservative and surgical treatment options, the patient opted for surgical correction of his painful ankle joint.

The patient's procedure was performed in the supine position and under general anesthesia. A thigh tourniquet was used for hemostasis. Incisional approaches may vary depending on whether or not a fibular or tibial osteotomy is necessary for exposure of the talar OCD defect. At that time, the ankle was exposed via an anteriomedial approach and all of the osteophytes, loose bodies, and inflammatory tissue were sharply excised. The medial osteochondral defect was visualized, curetted, and measured using a ruler. The octeochondral autograft transfer system (OATS) (Arthrex, Naples, Florida) then was used to make the circular defect in the talus. The appropriate small joint OATS set was selected based on the diameter of the defect. A guide pin was drilled into the center of the defect to 15 mm deep. The guide pin then was overdrilled with the appropriate size cannulated headed reamer to a depth of at least 12 mm. The cannulated OATS alignment rod was introduced over the guide pin for a depth measurement. This was tapped to the base of the drill hole for an accurate depth measurement. Once the dimensions of the talar defect were known, attention was directed to the harvesting of the autologous osteochondral donor from the plantar medial and nonarticular surface of the ipsilateral talus. In the presence of an accessory navicular, it is excised for better visualization and harvesting from the donor site.

A separate longitudinal incision was made over the medial aspect of the talus and over the talonavicular joint between the tibialis anterior and posterior tibial tendons. A longitudinal capsulotomy was performed into the talonavicular joint to expose the plantar medial aspect of the talar head. Care was taken not to transect the spring ligament. The appropriate size tamp was used to measure and determine the appropriate area for harvesting the autologous graft. Using the donor harvester in the OATS set, the osteoarticular graft was taken under fluoroscopic guidance to the desired depth. Care was taken to not enter the talonavicular or anterior subtalar joints. After removal of the donor graft, the defect was packed with a cancellous allograft according to surgeon preference. The wound was closed in a layered fashion. The donor graft was inserted into the recipient defect in the talus in optimal orientation for articular congruity. The white core extruder knob was turned in a clockwise direction gradually advancing the graft from the tube harvester into the talus. When the core extruder knob was fully seated the donor graft was slightly proud. The donor harvester was removed and the large end of the tamp, which measured at least 1 mm larger than the diameter of the donor graft, was placed over the graft. The donor graft was made flush with the surrounding cartilage by tapping it on the tamp with a mallet. At that time, if a small cartilage edge protrudes, it may be trimmed smooth with a scalpel. Range of motion of the ankle joint then is performed to make sure that there is a smooth gliding surface.

At that time and after the closure of all surgical incisions, the thigh tourniquet is deflated and the circular external fixator applied in a percutaneous fashion and with the use of intraoperative fluoroscopy imaging. The authors' external fixation system for the ankle arthrodiastasis procedure consists of a three-ring construct. Fine wires or half pins are inserted according to the lower extremity anatomic safe zones. Proper skin retraction and patient positioning are performed before insertion. The wires are tensioned with a dynamic wire tensiometer. Once the prebuilt circular external fixator is applied, the ankle is acutely distracted up to 8 to 10 mm. Intraoperative imaging is necessary to confirm the desired ankle arthrodiastasis and postoperative adjustments are made according to surgeon preference. One or two talar wires are applied and tensioned appropriately before the ankle distraction, which may be achieved manually through the external rings or the tensioned talar wires. In the case of a desired simultaneous subtalar joint distraction, no talar wires are applied to the circular external fixation. One to two midfoot wires also are applied for frame stability and assisting in the corrected foot positioning. An extra ring at the bottom of the footplate may be applied for protection at the first 1 to 2 weeks and is removed before the patient starts full weight bearing. Postoperative dressings and radiographs are performed every 10 to 14 days and the patient is encouraged to bear weight with crutch or walker assistance and after physical therapy consultation. The circular external fixator is kept in place for approximately 8 to 10 weeks and the patient then is placed in a removable walker for another 6 to 8 weeks. Postoperative physical therapy for decreasing any residual edema and increasing ankle range of motion is paramount to the patient's overall success (**Fig. 1**).

DISCUSSION

Growing numbers of patients are suffering from pain and disability associated with osteochondral lesions involving the ankle joint. Surgical treatments vary according to the size and location of the defect, patient age, and activity level. Over the past decade,

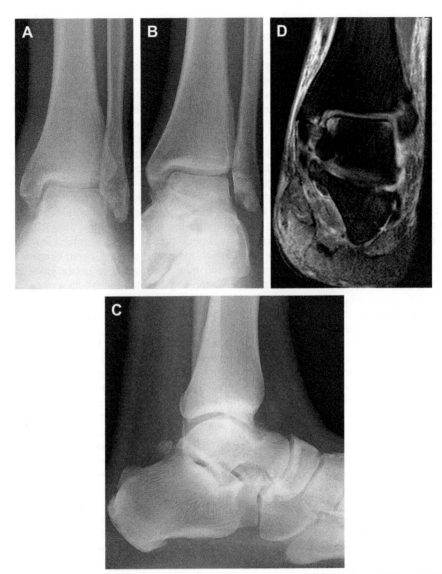

Fig. 1. Preoperative radiographic anteroposterior (*A*), medial oblique (*B*), lateral (*C*), and MRI (*D*) views showing the patient's symptomatic left ankle. Intraoperative view showing the incisional approaches for the simultaneous local osteochondral autograft and ankle arthrodiastasis procedure (*E*). Intraoperative view showing the OATS making a hole within the talar defect (*F*) followed by harvesting the autologous osteochondral graft from the plantar medial and nonarticular surface of the talar head (*G*). Insertion of the donor graft to the talar defect (*H*) with a final outcome (*I*). Note that the prominent surrounding donor cartilage is tapped on a tamp with a mallet or may be trimmed smooth with a scalpel to be even with the articular surface of the talus. Intraoperative views showing the ankle arthrodiastasis (*J*) and application of the circular external fixation (*K*). The bottom ring of the footplate is removed within the first 1 to 2 postoperative weeks and the patient is allowed to fully bear weight to his lower extremity. Postoperative radiographs at 6 weeks showing the ankle arthrodiastasis and alignment (*L, M*). Final radiographic (*N, O*) and clinical (*P*) views at 6 months' follow-up.

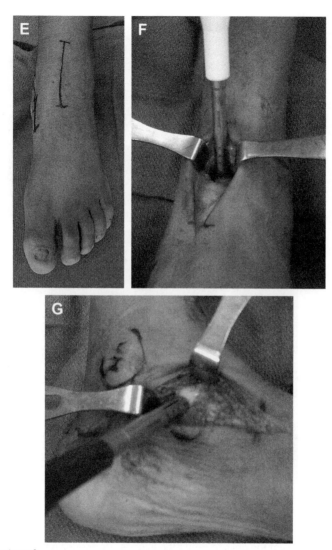

Fig. 1. (*continued*)

basic science research in the field of cartilage repair has expanded dramatically making the goal of cartilage repair a possibility.

Arthrodiastasis is shown experimentally and clinically beneficial in the treatment of ankle arthritis.[5–14] The theory is based on creating an intra-articular environment suitable for cartilage repair by ligamentotaxis. Chondrocytes depend on the diffusion of nutrients though a dense matrix for their survival. The cartilage vulnerability increases when there is synovial inflammation, loss of proteoglycans and collagen, decreased mineral content and density, and subchondral stiffness. Chondrocytes produce catabolic cytokines, matrix proteases that cause further degeneration. When the cartilage is damaged there is increased tension and shear around the periphery of damaged cartilage. Joint failure occurs when there is repeated mechanical damage that

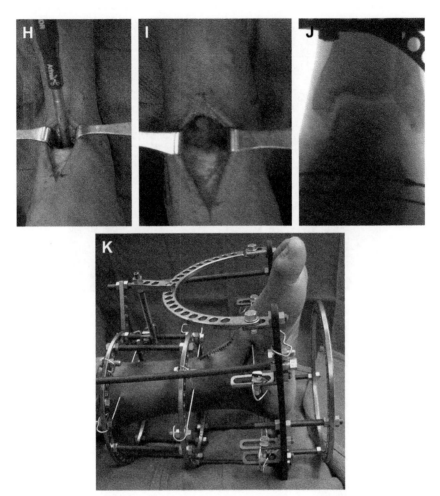

Fig. 1. (*continued*).

exceeds the capacity of the cells to repair the injuries. Rodriguez and colleagues[15] reported a case series of talar OCD lesions treated with transplantation of cryopreserved talar allograft and ankle distraction with a three-ring multiplane external fixation. All fixators were removed at 8 weeks and patients remained partial weight bearing in a removable cast boot for an additional 8 weeks. Radiographic consolidation of allograft was seen within 16 weeks. All patients reported a decrease in symptoms and improvement in levels of activity.

To the authors' knowledge, this report presents a unique approach not previously published for the treatment of larger talar OCDs by using a local osteochondral autograft combined with an ankle arthrodiastasis. This combined technique also can be achieved with the more traditional distant donor harvesting from the ipsilateral knee. Most common uses include but are not limited to younger, active, and compliant patients who have stage 3 or 4 osteochondral defects according to Berndt-Harty classification.[3,16] In addition, this surgical technique may be used for revision of previously treated osteochondral defects or as an alternate to ankle arthroplasty or arthrodesis.

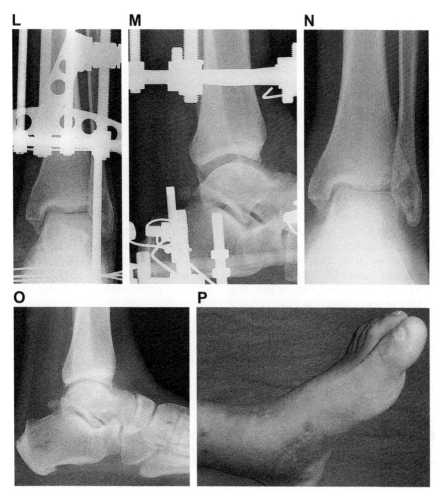

Fig. 1. (*continued*)

Contraindications for this procedure include infection, peripheral vascular disease, uncorrected residual deformity or ankle instability, neuropathy, and severe osteopenia. Relative contraindications include elderly patients, obesity, and smoking history. The advantages of this combined procedure are that it avoids two joint exposures, provides autologous chondrocyte transplantation, and facilitates the reparative process of chondrocytes to delay or prevent joint arthrodesis or total ankle replacement while allowing early postoperative weight bearing. The procedure entails open ankle arthrotomy with débridement, autologous local osteochondral harvesting, and transfer and ankle distraction by using a circular external fixation.

The authors believe that this method offers advantages to the autologous osteochondral transfer with early weight bearing and simultaneous ankle distraction to promote the reparative properties required for cartilage healing. The results of this procedure are promising in slowing the progression of joint degeneration and warrant further investigation with results from a consecutive series of patients.

REFERENCES

1. Buckwalter JA, Saltzman C, Brown T. The impact of osteoarthritis: implications for research. Clin Orthop Relat Res 2004;427:S6–15.
2. Alexander AH, Lichtman DM. Surgical treatment of transchondral talar-dome fractures (osteochondritis dissecans). Long- term follow-up. J Bone Joint Surg Am 1980;62:646–52.
3. Verhagen RA, Struijs PA, Bossuyt PM, et al. Systematic review of treatment strategies for osteochondral defects of the talar dome. Foot Ankle Clin 2003;8:233–42.
4. Sammarco GJ, Makwana NK. Treatment of talar osteochondral lesions using local osteochondral graft. Foot Ankle Int 2002;22:693–8.
5. Buckwalter JA. Joint distraction for osteoarthritis. Lancet 1996;347:279–80.
6. Chiodo CP, McGarvey W. Joint distraction for the treatment of ankle osteoarthritis. Foot Ankle Clin 2004;9:541–53.
7. Lafeber FP, Intema F, Van Roermund PM, et al. Unloading joints to treat osteoarthritis, including joint distraction. Curr Opin Rheumatol 2006;18:519–25.
8. Marijnissen AC, van Roermund PM, van Melkebeek J, et al. Clinical benefit of joint distraction in the treatment of ankle osteoarthritis. Foot Ankle Clin 2003;8:335–46.
9. Paley D, Lamm BM. Ankle joint distraction. Foot Ankle Clin 2005;10:685–98.
10. Paley D, Lamm BM, Purohit RM, et al. Distraction arthroplasty of the ankle—how far can you stretch the indications? Foot Ankle Clin 2008;13:471–84.
11. Zgonis T, Stapleton JJ, Roukis TS. Use of circular external fixation for combined subtalar joint fusion and ankle distraction. Clin Podiatr Med Surg 2008;25:745–53.
12. van Roermund PM, van Valburg AA, Duivemann E, et al. Function of stiff joints may be restored by Ilizarov joint distraction. Clin Orthop Relat Res 1998;348:220–7.
13. van Valburg AA, van Roermund PM, Lammens J, et al. Can Ilizarov joint distraction delay the need for an arthrodesis of the ankle? A preliminary report. J Bone Joint Surg Br 1995;77:720–5.
14. Zgonis T, Roukis TS, Polyzois V. Alternatives to ankle implant arthroplasty for posttraumatic ankle arthrosis. Clin Podiatr Med Surg 2006;23:745–58.
15. Rodriguez EG, Hall JP, Smith RL, et al. Treatment of osteochondral lesions of the talus with cryopreserved talar allograft and ankle distraction with external fixation. Surg Technol Int 2006;15:282–8.
16. Berndt AL, Harty M. Transchondral fractures (osteochondritis dessicans) of the talus. J Bone Joint Surg Am 1959;41:988–1020.

Index

Note: Page numbers of article titles are in **boldface** type.

A

Abrasion chondroplasty, for osteochondral lesions of talus, 212–213
Aggrecan, in cartilage, 171
Agility prosthesis, 303, 317, 319
Ankle osteoarthritis
  economic burden of, 169
  epidemiology of, 169
  pathology of, 199–200
  treatment of
    arthrodesis in, **259–271, 273–302**
    arthrodiastasis in, **227–244, 335–342**
    arthroplasty in, **303–324**
    arthroscopic, 212–213, **273–282**
    autografting in, **335–342**
    braces in, **193–197**, 262
    distraction in, **185–191**
    in end-stage posterior tibial tendon dysfunction, **325–333**
    scientific background of, **169–184**
    supramalleolar osteotomy in, **245–257**
    viscosupplementation in, **199–204**
  versus knee osteoarthritis, cartilage properties and, 175–177
Ankle-foot orthosis, 195–197
Anterior distal tibial angle, in supramalleolar osteotomy planning, 251–253
Arthritis, ankle. *See* Ankle osteoarthritis.
Arthrocentesis, for ankle osteoarthritis, 262
Arthrodesis
  arthroscopic, **273–282**
  subtalar joint, in combined procedure, for posterior tibial tendon dysfunction, **325–333**
  tibiotalocalcaneal, **283–302**
  traditional, **259–271**
    anatomic considerations in, 259–260
    diagnosis of, 261–262
    pathophysiology of, 260
    technique for, 263–269
    treatment of, 262–263
Arthrodiastasis
  clinical studies of, 232–236
  complications of, 236
  definition of, 230
  for posttraumatic arthritis, 228–230
  for talar dome defect, **335–342**

doi:10.1016/S0891-8422(09)00019-6
0891-8422/09/$ – see front matter © 2009 Elsevier Inc. All rights reserved.

Moving?

Make sure your subscription moves with you!

To notify us of your new address, find your **Clinics Account Number** (located on your mailing label above your name), and contact customer service at:

E-mail: elspcs@elsevier.com

800-654-2452 (subscribers in the U.S. & Canada)
314-453-7041 (subscribers outside of the U.S. & Canada)

Fax number: 314-523-5170

Elsevier Periodicals Customer Service
11830 Westline Industrial Drive
St. Louis, MO 63146

To ensure uninterrupted delivery of your subscription, please notify us at least 4 weeks in advance of move.

Printed and bound by CPI Group (UK) Ltd, Croydon, CR0 4YY
03/10/2024
01040444-0015

ELSEVIER